NO MORE W
STARVATION.
...GUILT...

NOW YOU CAN SAY GOODBYE TO
DIETING—ONCE AND FOR ALL!

"Jean Antonello's Anti-Diet Book reflects
all the new research on obesity. It tells you
what to do, how to do it, and why, based on
the *facts*." JoAnne May, Ph.D., psychologist

"The greatest thing about becoming
naturally thin, after actually *being* thin, is
never having to worry about your weight."
Mary Ann McTigue-Matheny,
businesswoman and ex-dieter

JEAN ANTONELLO is an obesity, eating
disorders and co-dependence specialist
at Passages Counseling Center, Minneapolis, MN. Formerly fat, now naturally
thin, she teaches classes and conducts
seminars, coaching individuals in obesity
recovery. She is also a well-known
speaker on co-dependence in the Twin
Cities area. Jean is married and has
three children.

Avon Books are available at special quantity discounts for bulk purchases for sales promotions, premiums, fund raising or educational use. Special books, or book excerpts, can also be created to fit specific needs.

For details write or telephone the office of the Director of Special Markets, Avon Books, Dept. FP, 1350 Avenue of the Americas, New York, New York 10019, 1-800-238-0658.

THE ANTI-DIET BOOK

HOW TO BECOME

NATURALLY THIN BY EATING MORE

JEAN ANTONELLO, R.N., B.S.N

AVON BOOKS 🔺 NEW YORK

If you purchased this book without a cover, you should be aware that this book is stolen property. It was reported as "unsold and destroyed" to the publisher, and neither the author nor the publisher has received any payment for this "stripped book."

To him who is able to do immeasurably more
than all we can ask or think or imagine.

My sincere thanks to Corrine Mady, Jeanne Hanson, Mike Beard, Joyce Hart, David McQuoid, M.D., Jeff Van Vonderen, Skip Billey, Fred Peterson and the Passages Counseling Center staff, and my husband Michael. Special thanks to all of the people who contributed to this book by sharing their experiences with me. This book is dedicated to discouraged dieters everywhere.

Before changing eating habits, you are advised to consult with your physician to discuss the proposed dietary changes. It is possible for certain individuals to initially gain weight on the Anti-Diet. There may be medical symptoms associated with weight gain for some people. Anyone experiencing symptoms is advised to seek medical supervision.

AVON BOOKS
A division of
The Hearst Corporation
1350 Avenue of the Americas
New York, New York 10019

Copyright © 1989 by Jean Antonello
Inside cover author photograph by John Bowman, Minneapolis, MN
Published by arrangement with the author
Library of Congress Catalog Card Number: 90-93554
ISBN: 0-380-76442-3

All rights reserved, which includes the right to reproduce this book or portions thereof in any form whatsoever except as provided by the U.S. Copyright Law. For information address Jeanne Hansen, 5111 Wooddale Avenue South, Edina, Minnesota 55424.

First Avon Books Printing: February 1991

AVON TRADEMARK REG. U.S. PAT. OFF. AND IN OTHER COUNTRIES, MARCA REGISTRADA, HECHO EN CANADA.

Printed in Canada

UNV   10   9   8   7

TABLE OF CONTENTS

The saddest thing
I think
Amongst all common but
Tragic ironies
Is to feel
Fat
and
Very hungry
At the same time.

JEAN ANTONELLO, 1974

FOREWORD

The topic of dieting often inspires emotional reactions, strong opinions, heated arguments, and intense despair even among dietitians! Dieters struggle with vague and contradictory information, destructive prejudices, wild and unscientific remedies, and many superstitious misbeliefs. In our culture dieting remains a hot topic because its traditional approach to weight reduction is destined to failure.

That's why we've called this book *The Anti-Diet Book.* It exposes two fallacies of the traditional weight-reduction diet:

1. People are overweight because they eat too much, and
2. People overeat primarily because of their emotions.

These approaches to weight problems are not only erroneous, they have perpetuated the problem.

This *Anti-Diet Book* deflates another common belief: naturally thin people are just lucky. In a way, this is true. Those who never again weight have managed to avoid the vicious cycle of dieting and overeating, but it is wrong to assume that they are the only ones, the favored few, who can enjoy freedom to eat. Anyone can.

This book describes exactly how an individual can be

forever freed from the traditional diet cycle and its devastating effects on the body and psyche. The freedom to satisfy hunger signals by eating real food is the privilege and responsibility of every individual, and it leads to a natural, adaptive, lean body weight.

How to Become Naturally Thin by Eating More explains how you can be permanently freed from dieting and overweight. It is a process. The process is not fast, but it is dramatic, particularly to those involved in it. Those who have never suffered from overweight cannot imagine the profound relief that those who follow this recovery plan experience.

This book exposes the real reason that people are overweight and sometimes eat too much. It teaches parents and caretakers how to prevent and treat overweight in growing children. *Naturally Thin* describes the true place that emotions have in the problems of overeating and overweight. *Naturally Thin* exposes the overwhelming physical cause of overweight and explains why people are totally helpless to overcome it without the new insights of the *Anti-Diet* approach.

Naturally Thin answers the painful questions that overweight dieters have secretly asked for years: Why am I still fat when I'm dieting most of the time? Why do thin people seem to eat and eat and never gain? Why do I gain when I'm trying so hard not to eat? Why do I feel out of control when I go off a diet? Why can't I stick to a diet? Why do I always gain lost weight back? There are answers to these questions. These answers will make real sense for a change, a permanent change in you.

MY STORY

Today, when I tell people that my book is about obesity, I almost always get a surprised look and this reaction, "You're not writing from experience!" They can't imagine me fat. Besides, I eat so much! I certainly wouldn't qualify as a good dieter! I act and look just like a naturally thin person. I eat anything I want whenever I want. I don't worry about my diet or my weight. My clothes always fit. I enjoy wearing a bathing suit. But it wasn't always so.

ADOLESCENT PANIC LED TO MY FIRST DIET

Like so many women, I started dieting in high school. After gaining a little thigh padding from hormones, I panicked. Thus began my diet history of over fifteen years. My weight fluctuated between 118 and 194 during that time, including pregnancies. Most of the time I maintained twenty to thirty pounds of excess fat. Maybe this doesn't sound obese to you, but I believed I was *very* fat, and I *was* very depressed.

THE THEORY OF ADAPTATION

After high school, I went to the University of Minnesota to study nursing. My love for science and people attracted me to the nursing profession, but my education alone did not solve my personal weight problem.

I learned much about the human body and mind with coursework in biology, anatomy, physiology, and psychology. But the focal point of my whole nursing education was the Theory of Adaptation. All the scientific knowledge I gained fit somehow into this fascinating concept of a human being's ability to adapt to diverse and changing environments. It was this Theory of Adaptation which would eventually lead to the answers to my own weight problem, but I saw no connection while I was in school or for some time afterward.

LOOKING FOR SOMETHING BETTER

Throughout high school and college I had tried to lose weight many times with many different diets. But five years after I graduated from nurses' training, I began to look for a better solution to my chronic weight problem. I was still overweight and dieting, off and on. By then I had had five years of experience in clinic and hospital nursing and was settled into the area of nursing called Medicine. "Medical" units in hospitals include most chronic diseases, including metabolism and nutrition disorders. Working as a charge nurse there, I had started to form some general theories and concepts about obesity but I was still far from a practical explanation or solution.

I WANTED A CURE

When my search for a solution intensified, I knew I did not want another diet. I wanted a cure. I wanted to be free of diets as I had known them. And I had known them most of my life. I longed to be naturally thin, but I believed it was impossible for me.

You see, I thought the world was divided into two huge groups: natural fats and natural thins. I was certainly a member of the former. It was so easy for me to gain weight, so nearly impossible to lose. How could I turn my heavy-duty body into a lean machine? Was it even possible to bridge that vast chasm between the two worlds of fats and thins? These questions motivated my research.

THE SEARCH FOR A SOLUTION

I started a small diet clinic where I shared my ideas and gathered more information. I read everything I could find on nutrition, obesity, and diets. I began to talk with people. I interviewed fat people, thin people, medium people, dieters, people who couldn't diet, people who couldn't gain, people who never tried, and people who never stopped trying.

REVOLUTIONARY CONCEPT

In all this interrogation, one particular concept emerged that revolutionized my ideas about obesity. It is this: Obese people, one and all, described feeling out of control during binges. They certainly wanted to be thin. They sincerely and persistently tried to stick to a diet. They had willpower. They were motivated by many important things—health, job, marital relationship, social acceptance, and self-esteem. In spite of these pressures and their own determination, they all reported that at some point in their dieting, something seemed to take over and sooner or later they went berserk—off the diet, on to eating. But never just normal eating. This post-diet eating was urgent, compulsive, excessive and out of control. It seemed that there was nothing they could do to stop it once it got started.

I, too, had experienced this many times. I began to think about it and gradually associated this experience with the Theory of Adaptation. In time, I concluded that the only force stronger than my desire to be thin (since that was my strongest conscious desire at the time), was my body's instinct to survive. This was the turning point in my understanding of obesity.

THE KEY: SURVIVAL

In school I had learned that survival was the compelling force behind the human ability to adapt to environmental changes. The instinct to survive has a very powerful influence on people as well as animals. It propels and motivates behaviors, even controlling them under certain circumstances. In other words, our physical drive to survive is so powerful that it will actually override our conscious choices if these choices threaten our survival.

In a way, our bodies sometimes take over the controls,

and we act or react on an instinct level. Under the influence of these powers beyond our will, we are out of control. Obese people, then, were accurate when they described feeling out of control during binges. And what was in control during these eating orgies? Their bodies, their survival instincts.

More questions followed. Why would the body provoke overeating in an already overweight person? What role does fat play in aiding survival? How does the body interpret the traditional food-restricted diet? With the answers came even more understanding. The puzzle pieces began to fall into place.

THE LAST DIET

As I applied the new insights to my own eating patterns, I stopped dieting. I began to listen to my body's signals for food. I began to eat more quality food more often, and I stopped trying to burn it off with exercise. The changes I experienced in getting off the diet/binge cycle were very, very gradual because it took me so long to break my dieting habits. I spent two years deprogramming myself (without guidance) from fifteen years of diet misinformation which had conditioned me to fear eating even the most healthful foods.

Inside, I still thought food made me fat. I kept trying to control my eating, off and on, and as long as I did, the diet/binge cycle kept going and my body kept my fat on me. Gradually, though, my weight went down as I improved my eating habits and eliminated my not-eating habits. Finally, I leveled off on the low side of the normal range for a woman my height. Unbelievable!

NATURALLY THIN

I have been naturally thin for over ten years. My body had the potential to become permanently and naturally thin all the while I was dieting, but I never gave it a chance. I wasn't eating well, and I wasn't eating enough.

After my third baby was born, it took my body only three and a half months to return to my normal pre-pregnancy weight. I had gained forty pounds and only lost eight with the birth, so three and a half months is quite fast. Many people, knowing about the baby, asked how I could have regained my slender shape so quickly. "I did it by eating a lot of good food whenever I had the urge," I admitted. They didn't believe me. By the time you finish this book, I hope you will.

INTRODUCTION

This Anti-Diet book is unlike any book on dieting that you have ever read. There will be no sample menus at the back, no chapter devoted to the caloric requirements of a moderately active homemaker or a sedentary businessman. There will be little talk of food restriction, either qualitatively or quantitatively. There will be no regimen to follow. In fact, there will be no diet to go on or off for that matter. No gimmicks, tricks, quick-loss guarantees or other promises.

What kind of a diet book can you have without calorie and carbohydrate limitations, exhortations, constrictions, promises, and sample menus? One that helps you to help yourself lose weight and stay slim permanently. That's the kind of book this is.

There are two kinds of dieters—successful and unsuccessful. The successful ones get thin and stay that way. The unsuccessful ones, 95% of all dieters, seldom ever get slim although they are constantly on a diet. With all their dieting, it's a wonder they don't fade away into nothingness. Why don't they? Because sometimes they're on a diet which causes weight loss, but just as often they are eating to gain.

Obviously, being on a diet doesn't guarantee permanent weight loss. This is the first misconception that has to go—the idea that a person goes on and off a diet. Actually, the very definition of a diet, as you know it, must change if you want to see any real change in yourself.

How can you possibly lose weight without a diet?

A DIET IS WHAT YOU EAT

By definition a diet is what you eat. It includes everything you eat, whether "off" or "on" at a specific moment. A diet is not what you don't eat. You are always on a diet, like it or not. You are either on a gaining, losing, or maintenance diet. It's not really something you can go off or go back on. As long as you think you go on and off it like a merry-go-round, you will be overweight, off and on.

If you can't go on a diet, what is this book about? It's about the basic definition of a diet: What you eat. 1. What 2. you 3. eat. What refers to food, all kinds of food, from celery to ice cream, lobster newberg to melba toast and everything in between. You refers to the unique individual reading this book—you. And, of course, eating is something you know all about, and also something you probably don't understand very well.

1. WHAT

Unlike many books on dieting, this book will not talk much about food. Although many would disagree, I have discovered that food is not the major problem for most dieters. I used to be afraid of food because I thought it made me fat. But food does not make anyone fat. It's available, period. It has no enticing properties of its own. Food does not lure, tempt, or demand to be eaten. It takes the blame from a lot of heavyweights because it is always at the scene of the crime. But food is an innocent bystander. It's just there, wherever you put it or happen to find it. You are what makes you fat, but don't start feeling guilty. Let's talk about you.

2. You

Again, unlike most other diet manuals, this book has a lot of information for and about you, the overweight person who wants to lose weight. Although you probably know quite a lot about yourself as a dieter, I am certain that you need some important insights to become a successful dieter. Most diets treat the symptoms rather than the disease, and most people go on diets in a temporary, just-to-lose-ten-pounds way. This book focuses on the whole person you are, rather than just the part of you involved in eating wrong and getting fat. Our goal is to de-emphasize the importance that food, eating, diets, and weight have had in your life because of your weight problem. As you grow smaller and smaller, your diet will mean less and less to you. Gradually, what you eat will take its rightful little place in your life. There are more important things to think about.

3. Eating

The topics of eating and eating habits have dominated diet literature. I will also cover this topic though from a new perspective. Diets have always been negative. They are usually written in terms of how and what not to eat. This is one of the biggest errors of the traditional approach from Atkins to Watkins.

I have discovered that if you want to lose weight permanently you must learn to eat: how to eat, what to eat, and very importantly, when to eat. You must eat in order to live. It's senseless, even harmful, to avoid eating.

But positive eating is only part of the solution. The key to unlocking your weight problem is understanding your body.

FAT AND SURVIVAL:
THE KEY TO WEIGHT-LOSS SUCCESS

There are forces at work in your body, beyond your control, which store excess fat. These forces are physical, not emotional or psychological. They are part of your body's survival instinct. As you read on, you will learn how and why your body works to keep you alive. You will learn the role that fat plays in your survival. Without an understanding of these things, you probably won't ever be slim for good. Armed with these insights, your chances for a new figure and a normal life are excellent.

What you eat, how much you weigh, and what your body looks like is largely your responsibility. I can give you direction, but you will be the one who changes you. No one can make decisions for you. No one can eat for you. No one else can make you a better person. But you can. Will you? You decide.

DISCLAIMER

Before changing eating habits, you are advised to consult with your physician to discuss the proposed dietary changes. It is possible for certain individuals to initially gain weight on the Anti-Diet. There may be medical symptoms associated with weight gain for some people. Anyone experiencing symptoms is advised to seek medical supervision.

CHAPTER 1
WHY DIETING IS IMPOSSIBLE

Hunger seems to be the number one enemy of the dieter. I say seems to be because actually it's the other way around. The dieter is the number one enemy of hunger. The dieter fights hunger in every possible way. She denies it, suppresses it, represses it, drowns it, and ignores it. You seldom hear a chronic dieter say, "I'm hungry. Let's eat." Once she commits herself to her new diet, it's down with hunger!

OVERWEIGHT DIETERS AVOID EATING

Hunger is not an enemy. Excessive hunger is, but that is the result of excessive food restriction. Everybody gets hungry, even the thinnest people. The main difference between the hungry thin person and the hungry fat person is that one eats and the other fights it. The thin person is the one who eats. She figures her body needs some food, so she eats something—automatically. The fat person who is on a diet already had her poached egg and dry toast for breakfast, and it's only 10:45 a.m. She can't eat yet because lunch is scheduled for noon. So she drinks a cup of black coffee, which is on the "any-time" list of her current diet, and waits until noon. It's a long wait.

VERY HUNGRY

Noon comes, finally. She is very hungry. The dry tuna salad isn't exactly her favorite, but it tastes fairly good. No bread. No mayonnaise. No chips. No Coke. Black coffee, anytime. She is gratified to have her hunger relieved. "It's working. I'm doing it!"

STARVING

At three o'clock she is mildly hungry. At four o'clock she is hungry. Her thin friend is hungry too and gets something to eat. Again the dieter fights her hunger. She made it to lunchtime, and she can hold on until supper. Black coffee, anytime. At five o'clock she is very hungry. At five-thirty she is starving and has a headache. She fixes supper, nibbling just a little, to hold herself off. She's almost there...

RAVENOUS

You know how the story goes. Ravenous by six o'clock, she eats supper and finds herself totally unsatisfied and still very, very hungry. She checks her anytime list for help, but there's nothing there for real hunger. So she begins to eat. She is going off her diet. She knows it, but she is terribly hungry. She is starving. She can't diet. She never could. She gets too hungry. So she eats. And eats. And eats.

She is stuffed, miserable, depressed, and fat. Hunger gets the blame, but hunger is not the problem. Not eating enough is the problem.

NATURALLY THIN PEOPLE EAT WHEN THEY ARE HUNGRY

Watch thin people eat. Invariably, they eat when they are hungry. They don't like being hungry, so they eat.

Dieters need to learn to eat when they are hungry, too. It seems so simple, but it has become a mystery. Dieters are so busy fighting hunger that they never consistently satisfy it. Then it turns on them and demands some attention. Eventually it gets some attention, too. Lots of it.

HUNGER ALWAYS CATCHES UP WITH THE DIETER

There are many variations to that story. I'm sure you have some of your own. Sometimes the hunger catches up with the dieter after a week. Sometimes after a month or six months. Whenever it does, the diet goes to waste. The dieter feels completely out of control and is. She did not take care of her hunger, and it came back to plague her, ruining her willpower and destroying all her courageous efforts to lose weight.

Some people never lose a significant amount of weight because of this problem. They are convinced that they absolutely cannot lose weight, no matter what they do. They are wrong.

A larger number of dieters lose weight by going on a highly regimented diet. Sometimes they lose a lot of weight. Losing the weight is not the problem. Gaining it back again is. When they regain lost weight, they are convinced that they simply slipped back into some bad habits and gained it back because of poor self-control. They are wrong, too.

Hunger and poor self-control are not responsible for the failure of the dieters described above, including you. Don't blame your body, and don't blame yourself. Believe it or not, your body works just like a thin person's. And until now, you haven't known any better way. Soon you will.

DIET ENEMIES MAKE SUCCESSFUL TRADITIONAL DIETING IMPOSSIBLE

If hunger isn't to blame for obesity, what is the stumbling block for determined dieters? Is it poor self-control? No. Excessive hunger is the #1 culprit.

DIET ENEMY #1: EXCESSIVE HUNGER

Excessive hunger is not a normal state. It precipitates such symptoms as headache, poor concentration, irritability, shakiness, palpitation, fatigue, and depression. Obviously, it is something to avoid unless you're masochistic, which I will discuss later.

Excessive hunger can be prevented by eating. There's no other way, and really, there's no better way. But dieters hate to eat while they're on a diet. They think that the less they eat, the more they'll lose in the least amount of time. Unfortunately, there are many bad side effects with this approach. Excessive hunger is the first and worst. Ultimately, it causes the dieter to fail.

DIET ENEMY #2: UNREALISTIC EXPECTATIONS

Most dieters think that if they eat sensibly they will gain weight, but they never really try it. They may start out that way, and in two days the scale goes up. "I knew it. I just knew it." they say. "See, I've gained. I can't eat at all without gaining." What they don't realize is that weight is not gained or lost permanently in two days. Two months, yes, but not two days.

This is an important point. The scale is not a god, sending divine judgment on your efforts to get thin. It is only an instrument which reflects general trends upward or downward. On a day-to-day basis, it is affected by salt-and-fluid intake/output more than anything else. You can't go by it. Perhaps month to month, but not day to day. The scale can help you, but you need to learn how it can and has hurt you.

DIET ENEMY #3: DIETERS DON'T KNOW WHAT SENSIBLE MEANS

Another problem for fat people who try the eating-sensibly approach is that they don't know what sensible is. Sometimes they have studied dieting so long that their notion of a sensible portion is actually far too small to satisfy their needs. Sometimes, because of chronic dieting, they find sensible amounts of food inadequate to satisfy their excessive hunger. And sometimes they come from overweight families where eating is never sensible. They habitually eat either far too little food or far too much.

These people need to learn when, how and what to eat from thin people, not from other overweight people.

But what's all this about eating sensibly? Is this the Anti-Diet? Partially, but there's much more involved.

DIET PITFALLS: WHY DIETS THAT WORK FOR A WHILE EVENTUALLY FAIL

Few dieters stay with a reasonable reduction diet long enough to lose weight. What's wrong with a typical diet?

First, the diet is artificial. It differs so much from the person's normal eating patterns that even after several months the dieter cannot learn it well enough to replace a lifetime of other eating habits.

Second, the weight loss seems too slow. The accompanying physical changes are not dramatic enough compared to the tremendous hunger and self-restraint the dieter must withstand. The compliments are scarce. The menu is dull. Consequently, she gets bored, tired of the suffering, and impatient for a size 10.

Third, the diet is not her own. Somebody else made it up. Somebody else doesn't have the foggiest idea about her hunger, habits, health, or home situation. She is not entirely responsible for her own weight loss as long as she is on someone else's diet.

Fourth, when her motivation is low and hunger is high, there's nobody around to help her get through, to build her sagging spirits, to bolster her courage. If there is a "supportive" person or group, they are as misguided as the dieter. They do not understand their bodies, even if they are slim, and they do not understand what causes bodies to be overweight.

Fifth, food is a source of fear. This factor is extremely powerful yet often completely ignored. The fear of eating is nurtured by traditional diets which support the fallacy that eating makes you fat. If this were true, controlled eating or eating less would automatically lead to thinness. We all know this isn't true either. The fear of eating is one of the most important obstacles to overcome in curing obesity. I will discuss this fear further in Chapter 3.

With such an array of obstacles, it's no wonder the dieter goes off her diet with more weight to gain, less courage to try. Let's consider each of these pitfalls separately.

DIET PITFALL #1: THE DIET IS ARTIFICIAL

If you want to lose weight permanently, you have to find a diet that you can live with for the rest of your life. It has to be compatible with your lifestyle and food preferences.

Ironically, it must resemble the way you eat when you don't consider yourself to be dieting. Of course, there must be changes in your usual eating habits, but if these changes are too drastic, you won't be able to keep at it permanently. You must start right where you are, adjusting your eating gradually and naturally as you lose weight gradually and naturally.

I can hear your protests. "Lose weight naturally?

There's nothing natural about me losing weight!"

Oh, yes there is. As a matter of fact, it's as natural as your gaining. Consider the natural law of energy. Energy cannot be created or destroyed, it can only be changed into different forms. If you take in more energy (food) than you use up, it will be transformed into stored energy or fat. If you consume less energy (food) than your body spends, it will be forced to break into the storage bins for energy, transforming the fat into a more combustible form and burning it up. Poof. You lose weight.

You may have heard all this take-less-in stuff before, but remember, the key is not controlled eating for forcing your body to get along on less food. That method almost always backfires. The key is to understand your body's needs and to let it use up stored fat as you give it what it needs.

Again, the chronic dieter's main obstacle is excessive hunger. She is too hungry too much of the time and little satisfied when she does eat. No one can live with that for very long. The artificial diet is to blame. It is not natural enough. It is not gradual enough. It is inconvenient. It causes too much discomfort and consequently can never be a permanent part of a normal person's life.

DIET PITFALL #2: WEIGHT LOSS IS CONSIDERED TOO SLOW

Permanent weight loss is always slow. A person can lose weight relatively fast, but then it is not permanent (unless there is illness). Permanent weight loss is always slow. Read that again. It's painful, I know, but it's true. You must believe it, accept it completely, and live by it before you will succeed at becoming a thin person.

In order to lose weight slowly you must learn to eat prophylactically, eat to prevent excessive hunger. You must eat when you are hungry and never, never get too hungry. Too much hunger is the enemy. Your body saves it up when you are not eating enough and then hits you with it at a vulnerable moment—a party, a vacation, or a disappointment. Feelings of hunger were never meant to be neglected. Your body's built-in mechanisms for survival will rebel. Starvation is not a normal state, but the chronic dieter suffers from semi-starvation much of the time. At other times she is eating too much, binging, out of control. What's a body to do? What are you to do?

PERMANENT WEIGHT LOSS MUST BE A COOPERATIVE EFFORT

You and your body need to get together instead of fighting each other. If you will begin to take care of your body's hunger, your body will begin to cooperate with your efforts to eat less. A paradox? No, it's logical. As you satisfy your hunger by eating properly at the right time, the distorted, exaggerated hunger you have forced your body to endure will diminish.

Gradually, you will begin to experience only normal hunger, which is not the enemy, but a healthy feeling. You will get in touch with the need for food. You will stop fighting yourself all the time. And you will eventually stop overeating. There will be no need. Eliminate overhunger, and you will eliminate overeating. Gradually. Slowly. Naturally. Honestly!

START BEING NICE TO YOUR BODY NOW

Your body can help you. It can be your friend. But you have to start being nice to it, even while it is still fat. If you hate your body because it is fat, you misplace the blame. Your body didn't make itself fat. The you inside your body did. You are responsible, but you have misunderstood your body. Blaming yourself won't help, and it may hurt a lot. Blaming, punishing, overeating, and obesity all go together. Diets and undereating link them together. You are beginning to separate them at long last.

DIET PITFALL #3: THE DIET BELONGS TO SOMEONE ELSE

A diet is a very personal thing by my definition. It is what you eat. It should never be what someone else has discovered that she can eat to lose weight. It's fine to share helpful insights about weight problems, but we are prone to trust in others' suggestions more than our own bodies. That's why, in counseling, I don't even talk about when or what a person eats unless there's a specific trouble spot to explore. Then the problem usually boils down to saved-up hunger, and we brainstorm possible approaches for the person to make a plan for herself. I don't have any idea what will work for her, but she does. And you do, too.

WE DON'T TRUST OURSELVES

We tend to trust others with our eating habits because we believe that trusting ourselves will cause overeating and weight gain. We definitely do not trust ourselves in this area.

Have we ever trusted ourselves and our bodies? Yes. When we were children, unless mother wouldn't allow it. We must have known something then that we don't know now. Or perhaps we didn't know something then that we have since learned that keeps us from trusting our bodies. What do children know about eating?

CHILDREN OWN THEIR DIETS

Around the age of two, most children become finicky eaters. They aren't hungry at mealtime. They want to eat at nonmealtimes. They don't like certain foods at certain times, and they won't eat them. They refuse foods that are purportedly good for them. They like peanut-butter-and-jelly sandwiches and milk and cookies. They like cold cereal and McDonalds hamburgers and french fries. And they *love* candy.

WHAT CHILDREN DON'T KNOW

There are a lot of things children don't know about eating. They don't know about nutritional requirements. They don't know about calories or fat. They don't know about dietetics, balanced diet, carbohydrate counting, or three square meals a day. They don't understand any of these things until we teach them, right?

WHAT CHILDREN DO KNOW

Children do know two things about eating: what they like and when they're hungry. They know what they like so well that they're usually willing to fight Mommy to get it. Of course, Mommy will work very hard to teach them that what she likes is much better than what they like. And as for their erratic hunger, Mommy thinks that if they had cleaned their plates at lunch, they wouldn't *be* hungry at four o'clock!

IF MOMMY ONLY KNEW

In general, children are in touch with their bodies, their physical needs. When they get hungry, they want to eat—in spite of the clock, in spite of Mommy's efforts to regulate them. They want to eat food that tastes good to them regardless of its caloric content or nutritional value. Feeding the children drives mothers crazy. And they often fight it throughout their children's grade school years. What's a mother to do?

While Mommy is encouraging "good eating habits" in her children, she is overweight, and they are slim. She is dieting, and they are eating. She is hungry, and they are snacking. She has two lean slices of beef and a salad, carefully skipping the baked potato and bread. They eat the potato and some bread, period. It's a riot. A sad riot.

OWNING YOUR DIET: NEEDS AND LIKES

Children own their own diets as much as we will let them. They eat according to their needs and likes, something they do know about.

The idea of owning your diet depends on two things: what you need and what you like. You can't ignore either without forfeiting possession of your diet and losing the weight-control game.

You probably gave up your own diet some time during high school, maybe earlier, maybe later. But when you did, you tried to learn how you *should* eat from someone else. You've had a battle ever since—a losing battle against gaining weight.

"Oh, my gosh," you protest again, "If I ate what I like all the time, I'd be even bigger than I am!" Perhaps you would, but I seriously doubt it. Regardless, I'm talking about what you need and what you like together. To regain possession of your diet you have to relearn what you need as well as what you like to eat. I'm certain you don't know either very well anymore.

WHEN YOUR DIET BELONGS TO YOU

Possession implies responsibility. As long as you are trying to lose weight on somebody else's diet, you are not completely responsible for the results. You can blame the diet itself for failure. When your diet is your own invention, you are making all the decisions about what and when to eat. You and you alone are responsible. You are forced to learn about yourself from your own personal experiences. You are forced to think about yourself, your eating, your hunger, your needs.

This is very important because you are the one who has overeaten and undereaten in your own unique way. You are the one who has eaten the wrong things at the wrong times. You are the one who gets hungry.

You make the decisions. You must change, for your-self. Until your diet belongs to you, you will always be fighting for control of your eating. Take control. Own your diet. It's yours.

DIET PITFALL #4: THERE'S INADEQUATE SUPPORT

When you start a diet, your interest and motivation are high. You are excited and hopeful. You are inspired by a fresh start. These natural positive feelings get us going in a new commitment, but they wear off fast. Even if you stick to a diet regimen for a longer time, the original optimism and excitement fades shortly after you begin. You adopt a milder form of motivation which unfortu-nately comes and goes. And your diet also comes and goes. And the extra weight comes and goes. How do you keep that motivation?

SUPPORT GROUPS CAN HELP

Support groups have become very popular because they work. They help people. In any endeavor which takes discipline, time, and feedback, the support of others helps. In weight reduction the support group plays many roles. It provides empathy for the struggling dieter. It provides reinforcement for accomplishment and advice for special problems. The support group can offer the dieter helpful information, provide a place for sharing, and promote confidence and friendship against the aloneness of dieting. The support group can definitely be an asset in weight control.

The type of support you'll need in your new approach to becoming slim is just as different as the new approach itself. The group (or individual) will still applaud your successes, but the definition of success will be com-pletely new.

The ultimate goal of the anti-diet idea is that you become slim and stay that way permanently with less and less effort until you don't have to think about your weight at all. It's a long process of learning about your body and yourself.

You'll need help in learning what your body needs when you get hungry, how you feel inside, when you need to eat, and what you actually look like. You'll need time, patience, and help. You'll need information that you can't get by yourself and compassion you can't give yourself. If you can't find a group, you will need at least one person to help you.

Groups That Don't Help

Traditional weight-control groups have a traditional diet style. They praise the person who has lost pounds (usually much too fast) as though it were a sign of success. Since permanent weight loss is always slow, this kind of reinforcement has unfortunate consequences for the chronic dieter. Inspired by her colleagues' applause for her five-pound drop, she goes home more determined than ever to lose and lose fast. With new determination against her hunger, she feels she is finally going to win. She's not.

Every person's body is different. Some bodies can tolerate semi-starvation for only a few days, some a week or two. Other bodies will take it for several months or a year. No one's body is designed to take it indefinitely, and no one's will.

A semi-starvation diet is any calorie-restricted or food-category-restricted weight-loss diet, frequently 800 to 1,200 calories a day or less.

The woman just described will lose weight as long as her body can tolerate her diet. She has always said she has to starve herself to lose, so that's what she does. She starves herself, and her group cheers her on. You know the inevitable sad ending to her story.

GROUPS THAT HURT

Not only is applause for fast, transient weight loss misguided, but the traditional diet group plays a destructive, judgmental role with its members. Confessions of binging and going off the diet bring sighs of disapproval from group members who have been "good" that week. Dieters fear weighing in without some weight loss to show, and they hear exhortations to get going if they have "only" maintained.

These tactics do not promote real success—slow, permanent weight reduction. They contribute to the chronic dieter's tragic cycle of weight loss/weight gain in fostering frustration, fear, guilt, and ultimate failure.

GETTING REAL SUPPORT

Learning to eat in a completely new way and learning to trust your body to help you requires a new kind of support group. (A group can be as few as two people.) As its name suggests, the group's purpose is to support the individual members in permanent weight loss and optimum weight maintenance. The group's role in the ex-dieter's difficult undertaking is vital.

In this new program of getting thin permanently, the group provides some of the same help that the traditional group provided, but the main emphasis is completely different. Traditional weight-control groups are organized to help overweight members lose weight. Most of the group effort is related to this goal, which is considered a fairly simple, easily solved problem: Eat less, lose weight. Eliminate ice cream, peanut butter, bread, and potatoes with sour cream, and lose weight. Simple. Too simple.

Because losing weight permanently is very different from just losing weight, the "permanent-weight-loss group" must be equally different. Goals and attitudes are different. Emphasis and effort go in a different direction. Most importantly, the results are different. They are positive and permanent.

GUIDELINES FOR A NATURALLY-THIN SUPPORT GROUP

The permanent-weight-loss group will remind its members of the facts about permanent weight loss—the all-important slowness of it, the natural plateaus in a gradual downward trend, the significance of owning your own diet all the way to your weight ideal, and the absolute necessity of eating to avoid excessive hunger.

The new group will reinforce new eating habits and eating attitudes whether the scale is momentarily up or down on meeting day. In fact, members will not weigh themselves in at all! The group does not judge but supportively helps its members explore problems that come up, offering alternative solutions for a person to consider and try herself. The group is a source of information and feedback for each member. The permanent-weight-loss group is truly a support group.

CHAPTER 2
STARVING AND BINGING:
THE FEAST-OR-FAMINE CYCLE

BENEFITS OF FATNESS

I have never read a diet book that said anything about the advantages or benefits of fatness. I have never heard a doctor or dietitian explore the possibility of a positive side of obesity. We have been taught, and believe, that a fat body is a body gone bad, out of control, self-indulgent. We are not about to consider the preposterous idea that fatness is a body's normal, adaptive attempt to survive. Taken to its extreme, this notion implies that excess weight and the ability to gain weight easily are good qualities in the human body. This is exactly what I am about to explain. Get ready, it's a very new idea.

ADAPTATION

What follows is not original thought. These ideas are based on the Theory of Adaptation, the central theoretical framework for the University of Minnesota School of Nursing, where I studied. The Theory of Adaptation proposes that individuals and species adapt to different environments in specific ways to ensure their survival.

The human body is built for survival. Its many complicated systems work together to ensure it. Some of these
systems are more easily understood than others, like the
fight-or-flight reaction to danger. When a person meets
with a life-threatening situation, the body instantane-
ously gets ready to survive. The pupils dilate, letting
maximum light in for more acute vision. The digestive
tract shuts down, allowing blood to circulate into the
muscles, ready for action. The respiration increases. The
heart pumps harder and faster, even before the physical
response begins. It's amazing and it works.

The human body has a tremendous capacity to adapt
to the demands of the environment. This is just one
example of our bodies' potential for adaptation. Because the human body is such a complex and sensitive
organism, the systems designed to aid our survival can
also create problems for us. They can backfire.

Just as we can learn how and why these adaptation
systems work to help us to stay alive, we can also discover
how and why they backfire. We often contribute to our
bodies' problems out of ignorance, false information,
habit, or a lack of discipline.

ALLERGY: ADAPTATION BACKFIRE

A good example of the body's adaptation system back-
firing is allergy. The body produces certain chemicals in
response to exposure to foreign materials from the environment. These chemicals, like histamine, help keep
the body clean and free of irritation and foreign substances. Histamine causes sneezing and tearing, cleaning irritant particles from the nose and eyes, and aiding
the body's efficiency and ultimate survival. The allergic
response to these same air-borne irritants is an exaggerated form of this normal survival system.

It's easy to see the logical purpose for the histamine

response and the important role that sneezing and tearing have in protecting the body from disease, but what does all this have to do with being fat?

HOW FAT GOT STARTED IN THE FIRST PLACE

Before people developed sophisticated methods for preserving food, there were seasonal variations in the availability of food, especially in cold/hot climates. Sometimes these variations were slight, but in extreme climates the food supplies changed dramatically from season to season. In order to survive the limited food supply, the human body, like that of animals, had to have a food storage system within itself.

During times of plenty the body had to be able to take in more food than it was using, convert this food into a storable form, and preserve it until the external food supply dropped below its survival needs. Then when available food was less than the body's current needs, it would slowly begin to convert the stored food into a usable, digestible form.

This pattern of preservation was as predictable as the seasons that caused it. Amazingly, our bodies can anticipate and make adjustments prior to an actual need, based on past needs.

Anxiety is a perfect example. Even before a danger presents itself, our bodies "get ready" for a possible threat. This readiness is important for our survival. But the response systems designed to help us survive often hurts us.

PATTERNS INSIDE AND OUT

The variation in food supply and consequent internal food storage system was indeed a predicable pattern. Human beings subjected to this pattern depended on their bodies' ability to adapt to these environmental changes. They ate in excess of their needs when food

was plentiful and stored the unused part for use later
when food resources dwindled. Because scarcity was sure
to follow plenty, overeating most likely began as soon as
extra food became available.

What does all this have to do with being slim? Everything.

By now you might be suspicious of the connection
between the last few paragraphs and your weight problem, and that's good. You'll need a lot more information before you understand completely. It will all come
together soon. Read on.

FAT *Is* ADAPTIVE!

Storing food in the form of fat is basically an adaptive
response. Your body is still capable of anticipating a
famine, causing you to overeat so you'll have something
saved up when you're starving again. The undereating
in famine times and the overeating in times of plenty are
intimately related.

If, like most chronic dieters, you are caught in the
cycle of starving yourself while you're on a diet and then
binging when your body can't take it anymore, your
body will never give up its fat reserves. It wouldn't make
sense. What if the next starvation diet or bacon-and-
grapefruit fad lasts as long as several months? How long
would a skinny body last? It's not adaptive to be thin if
you're dieting off and on. You need the extra fat just to
survive the diets. Are you beginning to understand?

Great. Our fat bodies are surviving the best way they
know how. Read that sentence again. It's true. Our bodies are doing the best they can under the circumstances.
What are the circumstances?

THE FEAST-OR-FAMINE CYCLE

1.   When you try to lose weight by the traditional
      approach, you do not eat enough food to cause a

slow, natural burning of extra fat.

2. By eating much less food than your body requires on a day-to-day basis, you impose a season of semi-starvation on your body. Your body "saves its hunger" (in the form of biochemicals, Ch. 9) until a time when it can overwhelm your dieting efforts and force you to overeat.

3. Since food is available to you, and the semi-starvation or famine is artificial (self-imposed), your body's adaptive mechanisms (survival instincts) conflict with your willpower.

4. Unless, by willpower, you work your way into anorexia nervosa, your willpower will lose the battle. You will not lose weight permanently. You may lose weight during the famine or diet, but you will always gain it back again.

5. Your body is convinced that your survival depends on maintaining a certain amount of fat reserves, and must carefully preserve excess fat and stay ready for a famine or diet.

6. Intermittently, your body demands feasts, which you also must reluctantly provide. You probably call it a binge or going off your diet. It's really a feast to prepare for and recover from the famines.

7. On the diet, you metabolize fat (and muscle) that has been stored during times of feasting (off the diet) and you lose weight temporarily.

8. When your body will not tolerate the fake famine any longer, it will force you to overeat to replace the lost fat reserves, converting the excess food to new fat. It is likely that your body will add new pounds of fat in case of a more severe famine ahead.

9. The cycle of feasting when you are off your diet and then starving when you are dieting perpetu-

ates itself. You are desperately trying to lose weight and your body is desperately trying to stay alive. It is an intense and extremely uncomfortable battle: You versus your body.

10. Your body always wins in the long run because its instinct for survival is stronger than your desire to be thin. Your only permanent loss is this battle against your body. You will gain and lose weight, but ultimately you will stay fat or get fatter.

No Exceptions

Every overweight person I have interviewed has confirmed that this cycle applies to her or him. Everyone can tell her sad story of weight loss and gain following this pattern. People everywhere are getting fatter by trying to lose weight! Despite their sincere and sometimes heroic efforts to win the battle of the bulge, they are ignorant of what they are doing to their bodies. They don't understand the principles of permanent weight loss. You are probably one of them.

FEAST-OR-FAMINE CYCLE STARTERS

During my search for the answer to my own weight problem, I conducted a class for dieters. It was a support group of sorts, but I was also gathering information from fellow dieters. During my initial interview with each person, I took a general diet history from her and discovered many interesting trends. (Note: Men usually have less-specific cycle starters. See Ch. 5.)

CYCLE STARTER #1: ADOLESCENT DEVELOPMENT

The most common age of onset for women is adolescence, often just after the first menstrual period. At the time they first considered themselves overweight, however slightly, these young women were also beginning to notice boys and to think about clothes and growing up. By the time they stopped to think about it, they already had a weight problem! Usually it was a minor problem, if a problem at all, but to sensitive adolescents it seemed huge. Losing weight took priority, and sooner or later they all went on a diet (more in Chs. 4 and 7).

CYCLE STARTER #2: PREGNANCY

Another typical Cycle starter is pregnancy. Women who enjoyed slim figures with little or no effort often complain that their first baby ruined it all. Actually, the baby didn't ruin anything, but the pregnancy initiated the Feast-or-Famine Cycle: feast during the pregnancy, panic after childbirth, famine to get back into shape, feast to stay alive (more in Ch. 8).

CYCLE STARTER #3: MOTHER KNOWS BEST

Other chronic dieters can't recall when they first realized they had a weight problem. As far back as they can remember, they've been fat. It seemed to start when they were born, but it didn't really. It started when their mothers taught them how to eat—according to her needs. They never owned their own diets. Their mothers started the Feast or Famine Cycle for them, often putting them on their first diets and cementing the Cycle into their little minds before they could choose for themselves.

This may sound a bit like an anti-mother campaign, as though moms are to blame for viciously and single-handedly producing obesity in their children. Although mothers do sometimes play a significant role, they are usually motivated by love and fear. Moms who are over-weight themselves have often suffered for years with the hopelessness of dieting unsuccessfully, and they are ter-rified that their children may be doomed to the same sad life. And so they erroneously conclude at the first sign of chubbiness that their children have inherited the problem.

CYCLE SENSITIVITIES

I will discuss heredity further in Ch. 4, but I want to make it clear here that although people don't inherit obesity per se, parents do biologically pass on to their children an "adaptation potential." To put it more sim-ply, parents whose bodies are highly sensitive to famines (diets, eating too infrequently, excessive hunger) often produce children with the same sensitivities. These more sensitive bodies readily store food in the form of fat in response to a decreased food supply (either real or artificial famine).

Some people have greater tolerance for occasionally going hungry. They are less sensitive to famines and don't gain weight easily. But highly sensitive bodies pro-duce overeating behavior (feasting) and weight gain with only gentle provocation (mild famines).

NINETY-NINE PERCENT

There are many other complex emotional, psychologi-cal, and physiological influences which influence eating behavior. I will discuss some of these later in the book. But I believe that the Feast-or-Famine Cycle of tradi-tional dieting is responsible for the vast majority of chronic weight-control problems.

FEAST-OR-FAMINE CYCLE STOPPERS

CYCLE STOPPER #1: EAT MORE

However you got started in the vicious cycle, there is a way to stop it. You must begin by learning to eat as though you have no weight problem at all, thereby eliminating the intermittent diet famines your body has had to adapt to. You will have to convince your body that it can safely stop storing fat. How? By eating well all the time. If you are coming off a restrictive diet, this process may take some time because your undersatisfied hunger has been saved up (in biochemical form) for the next feast. Going off your diet, even for the last time, is still your body's cue to overeat and replenish its fat stores.

So how do you permanently get your body to stop storing fat?

CYCLE STOPPER #2: EAT WELL

You eat. It's not quite that simple but almost. You eat whenever you are hungry. And you stop eating when you're full. Everything depends on the first sentence: You must eat when you are hungry. You have to show your body that food is always available in the environment. There is no need to store fat anymore. You can and must eat anytime your body needs fuel. Gradually, you will not be hungry for more food than your body needs at the moment, and you will stop overeating altogether.

When you stop overeating, your body will stop storing new fat. When you stop dieting permanently, you will permanently interrupt the Feast-or-Famine Cycle, permanently eliminating your need to overeat. And you will stop overeating and storing fat—permanently.

CYCLE STOPPER #3: KEEP EATING

Once you've interrupted the fat storage part of the Cycle, how do you get your body to use up the fat already stored? You keep eating. You continue to eat when you are hungry, and you stop eating when you are full. You must eat when you are hungry. Give your body a continuous supply of fuel, and eventually it will adapt to the new availability of food by lowering your appetite and burning unnecessary stored fuel. Your body will run at peak efficiency (positive adaptation) without the extra fuel-storage tanks.

How can you be certain that your body will use up the fat it has stored? How can you be sure that your body isn't just naturally fat in the same way that some people seem to be naturally thin?

This was my fear. But honestly, it wouldn't make sense. It's not in your body's best interest, which is survival, to carry unnecessary weight around. Eliminate the need by eliminating the traditional famine diets and— violà!—your body will naturally eliminate your fat.

Mine did. And I thought I was naturally fat.

UNNECESSARY FAT IS NOT ADAPTIVE

Excess fat on the human body is maladaptive (working against adaptation and survival) as long as there is a continuous, ample supply of a variety of foods in the environment. Medical science, psychology, and your own emotional experience confirm it. Obesity is maladaptive, undesirable, and destructive. In an environment of optimum food availability, it is a curse.

Your job in getting thin is quite simple then. Provide your body with a continuous, ample, varied supply of quality foods, and your body will do the rest. It's not as easy as it sounds, but it's easier than dieting. And it works. But there's more to learn.

HABIT AND WILLPOWER

There are two other important human qualities to consider. Both of these characteristics are built into us for adaptation and survival. But like the other survival systems, they, too, can backfire. One is habit. The other is willpower.

HABITS

Although the word habit usually evokes a negative reaction because of its frequent connection with the word bad, our ability to form habits is basically good and helpful. Good habits serve us in many ways, but we don't think about them because they are habits. A habit is something you don't have to think about. With so many things in life that we have to stop and consider, habits keep us from overloading. They are the brain's automatic pilot.

HABITS CAN BE CHANGED

Habits are learned, not inherent or predetermined. We are not born with habits, good or bad. The ability to learn new habits, unlearn old ones, and change our habits is inborn, and it is essential to becoming and staying slim. You have a weight problem partly because of your habits—your eating habits and your not-eating habits.

You might be thinking, Aha, here's the hitch. Right back to changing my bad eating habits! Hold on. This part is new, too.

IGNORING HUNGER MUST CHANGE

You don't need to put any of your bad eating habits in a straight jacket. In fact, you must not do that. There is only one habit you must change at first. That is the habit of ignoring, suppressing, or fighting your body's hunger. That's not difficult if you think about it and practice. In fact, after the initial shock, it comes quite naturally to eat food when you are hungry.

What about the initial shock? How do you begin to break the habit of ignoring, suppressing, and fighting your hunger? According to the definition, habits are automatic. You don't normally think about them. That's the key. Begin to break a habit by thinking about it. Think about your hunger. Learn to recognize it because sometimes it comes in disguise. Ask yourself if what you're feeling is hunger or a fuel-need signal from your body. Ignore whether or not you think you *should* be hungry and find out if you really are.

This may sound as crazy as the idea that fatness is part of a survival system, but it is a critical concept. People with weight problems often have no concept of their own hunger. They are so busy dieting or starving themselves that they have stifled their bodies' normal hunger sensations. Though not killing those feelings altogether, they have done great damage to their bodies' ability to sense and signal its need for food. The damage can be undone, but it will take time—lots of time, and lots of thinking. If you have damaged your body's communications systems, you will have to relearn your body's language. Listen to your body's signals and think about them. Learn how to respond to those signals. I'll help you.

WILLPOWER

The other quality to consider is willpower. Although habits influence our will, they can also change according to our choices. The will can dominate a habit and change it when we decide to change it, provided the habit is not essential to our adaptation (survival).

When you are hungry you are faced with choices. First you must decide whether or not to eat. If you decide to eat, you must decide what you will eat and how much. The normal decision is to eat something. The other decision is what will you eat? Notice the will in that question. What *will* you eat anyway? You have to decide that for yourself, but here's some information to help you.

WANT AND NEED

There are two things to think about when you are hungry and deciding what to eat: what you want to eat and what your body needs. Gradually the two will come closer together, but at first they might be quite different. Your ability to make wise decisions depends upon the intensity of your hunger. If you are too hungry, you will have a difficult time deciding what you really want to eat or what your body needs. Therefore, you must never let yourself get too hungry.

If you have ever looked at a big menu when you were starving, you know what I mean. All you know is that you want food and you want it fast in generous quantities. Your will is thwarted by your excessive need. In order to keep your will operating so you can make some wise eating choices, you must avoid excessive hunger. If you eat whenever you are hungry, your willpower can help you.

Oh, no. There's that awful word, willpower. You knew it was coming!

NORMAL WILLPOWER CAN HELP YOU BECOME NATURALLY THIN

There are different kinds of willpower: normal willpower and abnormal (superhuman) willpower. Normal willpower, which we all have, is the inherent ability to make choices. There's nothing mysterious about it. All it requires is an awareness of the alternatives. There is no pressure to influence the choice. There must be a choice to make in order to make one. If someone holds a gun at your head and tells you to hand over your money, what's the choice? You only hope you have some money to hand over! To have a choice at all, there can't be unreasonable pressure on either side.

ABNORMAL WILLPOWER WILL KEEP YOU FAT

Abnormal willpower is different. It is employed to enforce something that is contrary to our instincts. If someone had a gun at your head, and you had some cash in your pocket yet refused to comply with the demand, abnormal willpower would be at work. The chronic dieter employs abnormal willpower to avoid eating when she is hungry and food is available. It takes superhuman effort because she is fighting against the most fundamental drive inside her—survival.

By her will the chronic dieter creates an artificial state of famine and inflicts much discomfort on her own body in the form of unsatisfied or undersatisfied hunger. Hunger is painful. This response is completely unnatural because the adaptive response to pain is avoidance or withdrawal. If you touch a hot stove you will pull away instantly. A reflex does it for you even before you realize the hurt.

Unfortunately, the reflex is not as fast where hunger

pangs are concerned. Your body cooperates with your self-imposed starvation pain for a while, but you were never meant to ignore hunger when food is readily available. Sooner or later the will breaks down. When your body can no longer tolerate the suffering imposed by your will, it overrules your will and causes you to eat. You eat whether you want to or not. The survival principle is the most powerful natural force in you. Since your survival is partly dependent upon your body's avoidance response to pain (hunger), your body's instincts override your abnormal willpower in order to ensure your survival.

LEARN TO GIVE IN TO HUNGER

Abnormal willpower doesn't work in the long run, so you might as well throw it out now. Always give in to your hunger instead of fighting it. Decide to eat whenever you get hungry, and it will become a habit. You won't have to think about it anymore.

You might be thinking, If I ate every time I got hungry, I'd be enormous in no time! That's not true, but you will probably have to experience it before you can believe it. By admitting that you need to and will eat when you get hungry, you save a great deal of normal willpower for the important decisions that follow. Instead of exerting superhuman will trying not to eat, you can have plenty of willpower left to decide what *to* eat. What will you eat?

THE BIG ANTI-DIET DECISION #1

You have learned to want food that your body shouldn't really need. You have forced yourself to eat food you don't really like. You have refused to eat when you were very hungry, and you have continued to eat long after you felt full. You are overweight, and I hope you are beginning to understand why. But even if you are beginning to see the light, the question remains: What *will* you eat? I'm not going to tell you exactly, but I will share some important information that will help you decide for yourself.

DIET PROPAGANDA

Food prejudices abound in traditional diet literature: Proteins are perfect. Fats make you fat. Carbohydrates are the worst culprits. Sugar makes you sick. Saccharine is suicide. Grapefruit is great. Bran is best. The only way to be safe, it seems, is to go on a fast, and that really *is* suicide!

THE REAL SCOOP

I beg to differ. Proteins are pretty good. Fats are fine if few. Carbohydrates are OK. Sugar is special. Saccharine is sweet. Grapefruit is good if it's grapefruit you like, and bran is only better than a laxative. If I sound a bit facetious here, it's because there have been so many trends, scares, and revolutionary discoveries in the search for an answer to the obesity question. Medical training has helped me sort through these fads with some objectivity although I admit, I, too, have tried a few crazy diets.

FOOD DOESN'T MAKE PEOPLE FAT

In reality food does not make people fat or keep them that way. Certain kinds of food cannot be blamed either. People's bodies make them and keep them fat because of their maladaptive eating patterns. These faulty eating patterns create a physical need for fat accumulation that overrides all weightloss efforts.

REAL FOOD AND PLEASURE FOOD

I've divided food into two basic categories: real food and pleasure food. Real food might also be called need food because it's fuel for the body's needs. The primary purpose of pleasure foods is pleasure or taste satisfaction. These two classifications are general, and they can overlap. An English muffin with cream cheese and jam doesn't fit strictly into one category or the other. It meets legitimate needs and tastes great as well. Other foods, like ice cream and broccoli, fit more strictly into the need or pleasure group. But my purpose in separating them is not to label. That would encourage prejudice and unnecessary control in our eating choices.

What are the categories for, then? It helps me better communicate some essential ideas about what you are going to eat when you are hungry.

Good Taste

Everybody has different taste preferences, and these change from time to time. These natural variations in our desire for certain foods are important for several reasons. They help us select diverse foods, covering a broad spectrum of nutrients. Our desire for certain foods is likely related to our bodies' nutritional needs. Also, our changing appetites keep our diets interesting and satisfying as long as we are willing to adjust our eating to suit our appetites.

Traditional diets do not usually allow for the body's normal, dynamic food preferences. They try to make the appetite a static, boring, naughty child that needs strict limitations to force it back into line. This is wrong! Your appetite can help you become and remain slim forever.

THE THINK SYSTEM

THINK: What I Want and What My Body Needs

When you are hungry, think about your body's wants and needs together. You must not separate them because one isn't good without the other. Consider first what you want to eat, exactly what you are hungry for. Go to the refrigerator. What looks good to you? If you are not excessively hungry, you should be able to find something you want to eat. But stop! Before you eat it, think about your body and what it needs. If you have chosen a real food—say, a turkey sandwich—you can be certain that your body can use it well for fuel. It is a food your body needs and one that you like. Eat it and enjoy.

THINK AGAIN: Want and Need

Two hours later you are hungry again. Don't think about the fact that it's only two hours later. Your body is signalling the need for fuel and you will eat something. Back to the refrigerator or cupboard. What to eat? First, what do you want to eat? What looks good? Ice cream. Stop! What about your body. What does it need? What can it use well for fuel? Ice cream is primarily pleasure food. Right now you need to employ your will just a little. You're hungry for ice cream, but you're not convinced that's what your body needs. Does something else look good? A real food? Yes, a piece of toast with peanut butter and a glass of milk sounds good, too. Enjoy it.

THINK AGAIN: Needs in Disguise

But what if nothing else sounds good? What if the only thing you want is ice cream? Then stop and think a little longer. Since you're not ravenous, that won't be too hard. Think about your hunger for ice cream. Is there something else, something besides food that you need? Are you tired? Are you thirsty?

If your body doesn't really want the ice cream, try to figure out what it does want—perhaps a nap or a glass of water. If you feel OK, if there are no other needs imitating your appetite, eat the ice cream. You have not failed. On the contrary, you have won an important battle. You have accepted your natural appetite, but not blindly. You are discovering a new way of eating.

NEED MIXUPS

But what if you discover, and you will at times, that you want ice cream because you feel tired or thirsty or tense? First, don't eat the ice cream. It won't help you. Once again you need to stop and think. How can you help yourself feel better? What can you do, besides eating, that *will* relieve your discomfort? Drink something and lie down for a while. Get up and walk around the office. Call a friend. Clean a closet. Look at a photo album. Say a prayer. Do something to help yourself. You will feel better, and you will have beaten a bad habit—the habit of mixing up fuel needs with other needs.

Does this illustration imply that your hungry feeling wasn't really hunger at all? Yes, but don't feel too odd. Everybody gets hunger mixed up with other needs sometimes. Your job is to unmix them as often as possible. If you discover afterwards that you have eaten because of a need other than a fuel need, don't worry about it. You won't eat much to satisfy other needs anymore because you won't need to catch up on your undersatisfied hunger. Besides, this is all brand new. It will take a while to get used to. Take each hunger experience and try to learn from it. Gradually, you will find out everything you need to know to be thin, and you will be getting thin at the same time.

PLEASURE FOODS

There is a legitimate place for pleasure foods in your diet. You will discover what that place is as you go along. But you may surprise yourself at what you really want to eat when you are hungry. When you know you can eat anything you want, and you never have to put up with unsatisfied hunger again, it takes a lot of pressure out of your eating. You'll begin to want to eat what your body needs, and your body will begin to need foods that will lead to your slimness.

In the past, with all the famine diets, your body has needed fat-producing foods. These have been the foods you found most appealing. Now that the diet days are done, your body's needs will shift to lean-promoting foods, and your appetite will surely follow. You won't have to force yourself to eat or avoid certain foods anymore. Your body and appetite will begin to work together for a change—a change in you! You will want the foods your body needs, you will eat the foods you want to eat, and sometimes you will want ice cream. Then again, you might discover that you don't even *like* ice cream anymore! Isn't this exciting?

THE BIG ANTI-DIET DECISION #2

The quality of the foods you choose to eat is obviously an important part of becoming slim permanently. What about quantity? How much should you eat? How much of which foods is the right amount to get slim? How much is too much?

LISTEN TO YOUR BODY SIGNALS

Your body has all the answers and you'll need to start listening to it. At first, because you have abused your body's natural signals for hunger and fullness, you will have some trouble here. Just as you have to learn to recognize true hunger, you will also have to distinguish your sensations of fullness. Remember, habits are changed by first thinking about them.

LET GO

If you try to eat less than you want and stop before you are really satisfied, you are right back to the Feast-or-Famine Cycle. It's not a severe famine if you are eating some food when you get hungry, but it is still a quantity famine to your body. The food supply seems to be limited, or you would not leave your body undersatisfied. Your body doesn't care what's limiting the food supply. All it knows is what it gets.

GET TUNED-IN

You must learn to know when you are full. Not when you are almost full and not when you are too full. Learn to recognize the feeling of hunger satisfaction. Allow your body to tell you when to stop eating, listen to it, and then stop. This may sound like a gigantic hurdle, but don't get discouraged. You can do these things. They are natural, healthful, and easy things to learn. But they depend on your doing everything else you've learned so far. It all goes together.

STAY TUNED-IN

If you are eating something and you discover that you don't really want any more of it, stop eating it. If you are still hungry for something else, find out what it is, and eat that. When you are full, stop. When you want something else, change. It's so simple that it sounds ridiculous, except to the chronic dieter. To her it's a whole new ball game.

CHAPTER 3
YOU VERSUS YOUR BODY:
ENDING THE SECRET
STRUGGLE

YOUR BODY KNOWS HOW TO GET SLIM

You can trust your body and must if you want to be thin for the rest of your life. If you let go of the traditional diet controls and allow your body to adjust to the plentiful lifestyle we enjoy, you can trust it to gravitate slowly toward its most adaptive weight. All the evidence proves that your body's most adaptive, healthful weight is lean.

If you do not believe that you can trust your body and continue to cling to the controls by ignoring your hunger, picking foods you think are good for you, and forcing your body to adapt to an environment which doesn't exist, you will suffer a lot and never be thin. You will lose weight, and you will gain, but you will always be overweight.

YOUR JOB: GET OUT OF THE WAY

Your body can and will slowly metabolize excess fat through appetite, hunger, and hunger-satisfaction adjustments without your interference. Your job is to get out of the way and let your body work the way it was meant to work—efficiently, effectively, and permanently.

This theory is not a license to abuse your body by catering to your former ignorant whims, eating pleasure foods whenever the urge strikes. If you do that, you will gain weight. And don't tell your doctor that this book told you to eat whatever you liked, whenever you wanted to. My message is very different.

YOU AND YOUR BODY GET THIN TOGETHER

If you believe this Theory of Adaptation, it gives you permission when you are hungry to eat foods that you like and need until you feel satisfied. The theory not only permits this tremendous freedom, it insists that you learn to satisfy your body's needs in this new way. It opens a door between you and your body so that you can, together, ultimately fulfill your need to be slim.

I have purposefully not talked much about food because you probably already know a lot about food. But as helpful as nutrition information can be, especially if you grew up with unhealthy eating patterns, you can't start there because there's a real danger that you will begin to make decisions about when to eat, what to eat, and what not to eat according to knowledge rather than your body's signals.

WHEN WHAT YOU KNOW COUNTS

There are some situations where people must take their knowledge into consideration from the beginning. These are the exceptions, but it's important to mention them. If you have known medical problems—diabetes, cholesterol-related heart disease, hypoglycemia (abnormally low blood sugar), or any illness that involves your diet, don't be discouraged. This theory can work for you, too. The part you have to be careful about is what your body needs. In a way, you have an advantage over others. Medical science has discovered some guidelines you'll use to choose foods your body needs and can use efficiently toward better health. You have already learned some of your body's special needs that others will have to learn from scratch. Use these facts. They will help you become slim, too.

Just because your body requires some diet restrictions does not mean that you're limited in applying the theory. You can still eat foods that you like when you get hungry. However, the foods you like must also be the special foods your body needs. This will influence some of your decisions. But you are not up against anything that a completely healthy individual is not also coping with. Her body doesn't need an Almond Joy, either, right?

MEDICAL RESTRICTIONS

This paragraph always seems to find its way into diet books, and I guess it is inevitable. See your doctor. Do not try to explain this theory of permanent weight loss to your doctor. It's too new to you. Ask your doctor to read the book before you say anything about the ideas in it or apply the ideas to yourself (if you are medically restricted). Find out what your doctor thinks about your adapting the method to your eating program. Share your opinions. You should be able to work out something together.

❖

PERMANENT WEIGHT LOSS MUST BE PAIN-FREE

CHANGE—STRESS—PAIN

Change is stressful. Sometimes it is positive, sometimes it is negative, but change is always stressful. Stress causes the organism (human being) to make necessary adjustments in order to maintain life optimally.

Negative stressors, like cold weather following warm, cause discomfort or pain, forcing an organism to adapt or adjust. When temperatures begin to drop and daylight grows shorter, a horse's body, sensing the change, grows its winter coat. When the fall chill hits us, we get our parkas out of the attic. So, change is stressful. And stress is, in a way, always painful. Therefore, change is painful.

CHANGE AVOIDANCE IS ADAPTIVE

Since the adaptive response to pain is avoidance and change involves discomfort or pain, it follows that healthy organisms would tend to avoid change. And they do. It's an adaptive quality.

You must be wondering by now what all this has to do with thinness. The key is gradual change. In order to eliminate the stressful and hence painful elements of change, body weight changes must occur so slowly as to be imperceptible on a day-to-day basis. Without the stress and consequent pain of sudden, perceptible change, your body's natural tendency to resist is eliminated. And so it allows gradual, necessary, adaptive adjustments in your weight.

SUFFERING TO LOSE WEIGHT DOESN'T HELP. IT HURTS

The point is that you should not suffer, at least not perceptibly, while you are losing weight. It is not adaptive to inflict pain on yourself, even in the cause of getting thin. There's the rub.

You may be convinced that you must endure suffering in order to lose weight. You must pay for your sins of overindulgence. Wrong. The exact opposite is true. You must not and indeed cannot lose weight permanently by forcing your body to withstand the pain of unsatisfied or significantly undersatisfied hunger. There's too much inherently working against your survival instincts and your body can't afford to cooperate for very long.

WHY MORNING FAMINES ARE MOST POPULAR

These ideas have helped me to understand why so many dieters do their dieting early in the day. This is so common that it warrants explanation. Remember the story about the woman at the beginning of the book who managed to stay with her prescribed reduction diet fairly well until evening? She is a good example of the problem I'm talking about.

First, because of the false belief that she must endure the pain of hunger in order to lose weight, she did not eat much until long after she was just hungry. Second, when she did eat, she ate way too little food, leaving her exaggerated hunger undersatisfied and her body uncomfortable just a short time later. Her willpower battled her hunger, and her willpower managed to win, for a while. She had to employ lots of abnormal willpower in her attempt to lose weight this way, but she wanted so desperately to lose the ugly fat that her will was strong, stronger than her body's need—until evening.

What went wrong then? What broke her determined will later that night? Surely it was not lack of motivation or sincere desire. She had wept about her fat body. We've ruled out a weak will. She needed superhuman discipline to resist her natural survival instincts. What then? Let's go back to pain, stress, and change.

If change is stressful and stress is painful, then change is painful. And trying to lose weight by going hungry causes an adaptive resistance in the body. Hunger is a pain the body naturally eliminates. To tolerate such pain unnecessarily requires excessive willpower, but such powers of the human will exist where desire is very high.

This explains what happened to the woman in the story before suppertime. But why did she give up then? I believe it was the extreme hunger plus fatigue plus having to fix dinner plus depression about being fat. These are all sources of stress and pain. The heart is willing but the body is not weak. Its drive to survive wins in the end. Sometime you'll be grateful for that.

The woman in the story was not grateful. She started down the familiar road of overeating, perplexed about the whole thing. She was fighting a losing battle with her own body, feeling guilty all the way.

WHEN AND HOW THE BODY BURNS UNNECESSARY FAT

If you must avoid the perceptible pain of hunger in order to lose weight permanently, when does your body get a chance to metabolize your excess fat? If, whenever you get hungry, you eat until you are completely satisfied, when does your body use up its fat stores? When can your body get empty without feeling hungry? My guess is during the night. Although I've never read any scientific studies to prove it, I've made several observations that support this possibility.

EATING PATTERNS SHIFT

The people who have applied this theory persistently have reported an interesting shift in their eating habits even within the first weeks. They change from morning dieters to morning eaters and their nighttime binges stop effortlessly. They say, and I have also experienced this, that they seem to be more hungry more often in the early part of the day, so naturally, they eat more then. As they keep their hunger satisfied, their appetites dwindle, which is just the opposite of the chronic dieter just discussed.

Often, they report, they eat a last meal around four or five o'clock, and that's the last time they feel really hungry. Before bed they have a pleasant feeling of emptiness but often they do not feel hungry or desire food. So they do not need to eat then. They grow hungry during the night, I presume, but because they're asleep they don't feel it. Without ready calories available from the outside, their bodies quietly shift to using stored calories, and their fat is metabolized.

Since imperceptible hunger pain does not provoke the body's resistance, the battle with the body never begins. As soon as they feel the discomfort of hunger after waking, they eat a satisfying breakfast. Breakfast literally means to break a fast, a nighttime fast.

This example does not imply that you should go to bed hungry, or that you shouldn't have a meal after five o'clock. I sometimes eat a plate of spaghetti with toast before bed because I'm hungry for it. But I usually eat so well all day, I don't *want* food at night.

HUNGRY SLEEPING BABIES

I've also found support for this hypothesis in observing my newborn baby. When Genevieve was three months old, she was on a demand feeding schedule. She usually fell asleep at seven or eight o'clock in the evening. Since I was up until about twelve and knew she wouldn't sleep through till morning, I would wake her for a feeding. She was sound asleep at midnight, apparently perfectly content. It always took a few minutes on the changing table before she was fully awake, but once awake, she was *hungry*! She was very hungry and cried vehemently if I put her off.

Ten minutes earlier she was blissfully asleep, but once awake, she would be in real pain, and her body would not tolerate it for long. Her body is not built to tolerate pain. On the nights I let her sleep through my bedtime she usually slept until about four a.m. before waking to eat. This implies that she was experiencing imperceptible hunger pain for at least four hours on those nights that I didn't feed her at twelve. And what do you suppose her little body was using for fuel during all that time? Right. Fat.

BLOOD SUGAR EFFECTS

There's one other factor to consider in this nighttime weight-loss idea: blood sugar level. It's important for you to know that activity has an effect on the level of ready energy fuel (sugar) in your blood, especially if you haven't eaten for a while. Your body uses up some of the sugar in your bloodstream during physical activity so that as you exert yourself, your blood-sugar level falls. This is normal. When it falls to a certain level, your body begins to signal a need for more fuel. Your liver does some extra work. Your pancreas does some, too. Many intricate systems in the body work hard to ensure an adequate level of sugar in your blood during activity.

After you stop exercising and rest awhile, you may begin to feel hungry. This is a signal that the fuel you've used needs replacing. When the hungry feeling is delayed a few hours after exercise, the body's internal systems are holding the blood sugar within normal limits without fuel. Many exercisers experience this hunger delay or suppression with increased activity. It is a healthy, adaptive response. (More on exercise in Ch. 5.)

During the night when you are asleep, the chain of events, which maintains a normal blood-sugar level during activity, does not occur. There is no significant physical exertion to start it. What about the blood-sugar level then? Instead of dropping in response to the activity and going back up as the various systems work, it is steady during sleep. Changes are very gradual. The body can keep a fairly constant, normal blood-sugar level while you are at rest, like a well-tuned engine in neutral. The RPMs don't change, even though the motor is on.

So what? If your blood-sugar level is steady, and your body is maintaining a normal level of ready fuel, the sensation of hunger that you sometimes feel after activity will not occur during the night while you are at rest. Although the changes your body makes to break down fat cells for fuel is somewhat stressful for the body, other stressors are not present at complete rest, or they are imperceptible. There is no additive effect as there was in the story of the woman who went hungry until suppertime, then went crazy. What better time for your body to metabolize extra fat than during the night while you sleep? That's when other stresses are minimized.

EMERGENCY FAT: STRANDED WITHOUT FOOD

There will be other times when your body will naturally call upon its fat reserves for needed fuel. You have to be careful here because there's room for misunderstanding. I refer to those occasions when you get hungry and there really is no food available to you for a time. I say occasions because I trust that, having learned about your body's ways, you will do your best to keep them occasional.

When you are caught hungry without a source of

food, your body will begin to use some of its stored fuel, glycogen, for its needs. Glycogen storage is one of the important functions of the liver. Your body's fuel-supply systems will change gears from metabolizing food to breaking down glycogen into a usable energy form, either glucose or sugar. One of the reasons you feel hungry is your falling blood-sugar level. And once again these systems work to keep that level within healthy limits. This explains why sometimes, after you experience hunger pangs, your hungry feelings seem to go away. Don't be fooled, though. As soon as you have the opportunity to eat, eat.

HELP! NO REAL FOOD AVAILABLE

Suppose you get unexpectedly hungry during a meeting or in class and once you adjourn, you're hungry for a sandwich, but all that's available in the vending machine is candy bars. You know your body doesn't need a candy bar, right? Wrong. In this situation your body needs fuel, any usable fuel, and a candy bar is fuel. You may not even want a candy bar, but your body's need takes precedence over what you want at this point. So pick a candy bar, one with nuts or seeds if you like them, and eat it. You will feel better, at least temporarily.

REAL FOOD ASAP

Candy bars are mainly pleasure foods, but, as the example shows, they can serve as real foods, too. Because pleasure foods are usually qualitatively different from real foods, when you have to substitute one for the other like this, you'll need to get some real food to eat as soon as you can. It's not wise to wait until you're really hungry again either, because your hunger, temporarily put off by a substitute food, will probably come back very strong. Strong hunger is excessive hunger, and excessive hunger is the enemy. So as soon as you have a chance, eat some real food for your body's sake. And don't worry about the candy bar. It served a good purpose.

"MALIGNANT DIETITIS"

If you get hungry in a vending machine situation like this and you don't have any money, borrow some. Tell the lender you have an illness. Call it dietitis or something, and explain that when you get hungry, you absolutely must eat. If you don't, you'll grow faint and irritable and eventually get very fat! The lender won't refuse your request. If she doesn't have the change you need, she'll get it for you! Or maybe she'll share her lunch.

TO LOSE EMERGENCY FAT, BE PREPARED

To prevent having to eat food you don't want or don't need, anticipate your hunger and prepare for it. Learn about your body's fuel needs. Find out how long a bowl of cold cereal with toast and juice will actually hold you before hunger sets in. If it's one hour, fine. Figure out where you'll be when that meal is all used up. If there won't be any real food there that you'll want, take something with you. When you have just eaten a satisfying meal, it is difficult to imagine your next hungry feelings. But you must remember that you usually get hungry after a while. Act beforehand on that knowledge. You *will* get hungry again, sooner or later.

Sandwiches and fruit are just as portable as granola bars, and your body probably needs more of the former. Don't worry about the bread in a sandwich, either. Bread is a great, delicious, nutritious, and convenient food. You may eat it in good health whenever and wherever you are hungry for it. Isn't this fun? (More on bread in Ch. 4.)

BE PREPARED: KEEP REAL FOOD AVAILABLE

The availability of real foods is an extremely important point. If you get hungry after a coffee party, and you have a big tray of coffee cake left and nothing else to eat that has any appeal, your body will be inclined to accept the coffee cake for fuel. Coffee cake is essentially a pleasure food and a poor substitute for real food. You know your body doesn't need coffee cake because you are really hungry for scrambled eggs or quiche. You have set yourself up to eat pleasure food inappropriately.

It is far from ideal to eat coffee cake in this situation because you want and need real food. You could have kept your real food supply handy, but you are stuck with the coffee cake because real food is not available. The moral of the story is this: keep a plentiful stock of real foods, foods you like and foods you know your body needs for fuel.

PLEASURE FOODS

When are pleasure foods appropriate, then? Good question.

Desserts are almost always pleasure foods, and pleasure foods are often sweet. Even fruit can pass for pleasure purposes. It has become a popular dessert food recently. Why did the tradition of eating sweet pleasure foods after a meal come into our culture? The reason we create and continue with certain cultural habits is that they serve practical and/or logical purposes. Our bodies communicate their needs and appetites in a general way through these trends.

The waitress smiles. "Would you like dessert tonight?"

You are already satisfied. You know you are. But something about that question appeals to you. Can you trust yourself? Last night you absolutely did not want dessert, and you knew that, too. Can you trust this feeling, this craving? Is this hunger? Yes, it's a form of hunger, and there are good reasons behind it.

WHY DESSERTS ARE SO APPEALING ... TO EVERYONE

After a meal, your body goes to work to change the food you have just eaten into a usable form. This takes energy, and the blood circulating in your body carries this energy to your digestive tract where it is used to digest food. You might feel tired or more relaxed after eating a meal, especially a heavy one, because of this shift. Your body is using the most available form of fuel, sugar, to digest new fuel for eventual use. So what happens to the level of sugar in your blood? It drops temporarily, even though you have just eaten a meal. You have a vague desire, even a craving for something that will quickly bring your blood-sugar level up again. This something should not take too much digestive energy to get into the bloodstream, and it should provide quick fuel against the sluggish feeling you have. You want something sweet, something with sugar, honey, or the natural sugar—fructose. Pleasure foods are usually sweet, and desserts are pleasure foods, so you want a dessert-type food.

Teas and coffee also often follow a meal, and I suspect it's for the same reason. They help perk you up from the tired feeling you get after you eat. Besides, they do go so well with sweets!

HOW MUCH FAT CAN YOU LOSE NATURALLY?

Perhaps the most important question you have is still unanswered. According to this Adaptation Theory, how much weight should your body naturally burn up? The answer is fairly simple. Your body will lose as much fat as necessary to work at peak efficiency given its environmental food supply. In a way then, since you provide the food available to your body, the amount of weight you will adaptively lose depends largely on you.

It does not depend on how hard you try to diet or control your eating. It depends on how well you use the variety of high quality foods that you have. By your provision of good food, you will allow your body's normal, adaptive leanness to evolve. Your body will burn excess fat, which you have made unnecessary in this new environment of abundance. Only a small, healthy amount of fat will remain. You will be thin for good.

THE FAT YOU KEEP

What about this small, adaptive amount of fat that you keep? Let's discuss the situation for men here. (For the special fat that women keep, see Ch. 6.)

Why should older men have less need of fat than younger men? This is an oversimplified generalization, so I will give an overly simple, general answer: differences in activity level or exercise. Usually, older men, especially after retirement, are less physically active than their younger counterparts, who are still going to jobs and keeping busy with family and/or vigorous sports. This is not to say that many older men are not as physically fit as the younger. The opposite is often true. Older men who are more conscious of their bodies' needs for physical activity and have more time, may pursue regular physical exercise. Feeling great doesn't come as easily to them, perhaps, as to the younger men, so they determine to work at things that help them feel great. Exercise is one of those things.

Generally, younger men are more physically active. Why then, should they need more fat? More activity, more fat? Less activity, less fat? That doesn't seem to make sense. You always thought it was the other way around, right? There are a lot of things in this book that you thought were the other way around. But fat and exercise do go together.

Let me first make it clear that I am talking about small, adaptive amounts of fat on a physiological, cellular level. As a rule, athletes are not supposed to look fat. They need to have more fat than sedentary nonathletes do, but that fat is well hidden in the extra musculature of their bodies.

ACTIVES AND SEDENTARIES

Let's reclassify the groups by level of physical activity alone instead of older and younger, men or women. Now we have two basic categories of people: sedentaries and actives. We all fit into one of these categories or somewhere in between. Other variables aside, sedentary bodies need less fat (on a cellular level) for efficient adaptation to the environment than more active bodies do. The actives need and have more hidden fat.

OVERWEIGHT PEOPLE NEED THEIR EXCESS FAT

The problem you might be having with this idea is related to the maladapted, obese, sedentary body. It seems that the slower you go, the fatter you get. But my concept about active versus sedentary fat requirements cannot apply to such a body. I have already explained why people get fat and stay that way, and it has little to do with exercise in my opinion. The obese body acquires and keeps its fat because of an artificial need to make up for famine dieting or reckless eating habits.

This is the first time in the book that I've mentioned exercise, so try for a moment, to forget everything you've ever heard about exercise and weight control.

FAT IS SURVIVAL INSURANCE

Because the energy requirements of an active body are generally higher than those of a sedentary one, the active body needs to maintain larger stores of internal food supply in case of lowered food availability. This is true even if there are no real or artificial famines imposed on these bodies because the body is constantly ready for the possibility that food will sometime be unavailable. If stranded in the desert without food, the denser, muscular body of the active person would burn more stored fuel faster than the nonmuscular, sedentary person's. Because of their different energy needs, they require differing amounts of stored fuel to ensure survival.

HEALTHY SEDENTARIES NEED LESS FAT

In their most adapted condition, then, the sedentaries need less fat. Their bodies work most efficiently on the very lean side.

Consider the difference between Olympic women skaters and fashion models. The skaters are meatier, fuller-bodied women, and that's not all muscle. Less athletic fashion models who are naturally very slim sometimes have a problem keeping their weights up. Their bodies do not have a need for more than a minimal amount of fat and muscle because their activity level is not as high as the professional athlete. These bodies are well adapted to environments where exercise has its influence, but eating patterns determine fat needs much more than exercise does.

EXERCISE AND WEIGHT PROBLEMS

This connection between fat, muscles, and exercise does not mean that you should not exercise! It does have some implications for actives and sedentaries with weight problems.

SEDENTARY OVERWEIGHTS

First, the nonactive overweights. You needn't change your activity level in order to be slim. I have found that exercise programs for naturally sedentary people are often artificial and temporary. They also add stress to an already stressful diet. If you persist in eating according to your body's needs and signals, your body will adjust itself and your weight to the amount of activity that's natural for you. I believe it is harder on your body to start and stop various exercise programs than it would be to simply accept your nonactive lifestyle. Exercise alone will not make sedentaries thin. Exercise does have many benefits for you and your body (see Ch. 5), but only eating right will lead to your thinness.

ACTIVE OVERWEIGHTS

Those who maintain a relatively high level of physical activity day to day need to remember that the body stores fat because of its needs. If you have a weight problem which is caused by the Feast-or-Famine Cycle, you may be adding to your body's need for fat by your high activity level and/or exercise program. That's ironic, isn't it? But it is possible. It does not mean that you should cut down on activity or stop exercising!

But, as you break out of the cycle of undereating and overeating, eliminating your body's greatest need to store fat, you will still have a significant, legitimate need for a supply of extra muscle fat. Remember, this is not fat that shows. It is hidden in the muscle tissue. This true-fat need may influence the rate at which your body gives up its extra, unnecessary fat stores. It may slow it down. Consequently, the athlete, once off the Feast-or-Famine Cycle, may lose weight a little more slowly than the spectator who breaks the Cycle. But maybe not. Every body is different.

If this happens to your athletic body, you'll know what's behind it. Of course, individual differences in metabolism and degree of obesity will also have a decided effect on rate of weight loss.

WELL-CONDITIONED WRESTLER

The year after I was married, I gained 20 lbs. (Of course, this followed a 20 lb. weight loss before my wedding.) I was very depressed about my weight and equally determined to do something about it. I had tried everything eat-less diet literature had to offer, and I was desperate. That's why Dr. Atkins' promises appealed to me. I had to lose weight, and he said I would, eating as much as I wanted! (I'll get back to Dr. Atkins' Diet later on, but right now the story is more important.)

I swore off carbohydrates completely. That's the way you start the Atkins Diet Revolution. You stop eating anything with carbohydrates in it: bread, potatoes, fruit, vegetables, milk, ketchup, and all sorts of other horrible foods. (You may detect a note of sarcasm here. It was a terrible experience.) Dr. Atkins said these foods were to blame for making me fat, and I believed him. I was desperate.

Because I was so determined, I coupled my anti-carbohydrate regimen with regular, vigorous exercise. I ran several miles every day, sometimes twice a day. I did floor routines, too. Dr. Atkins did tell me one good thing. He told me I could eat whenever I was hungry. So I did. But I did not eat the foods I like or those my body necessarily needed. I ate only meat, fish, poultry, and eggs. I dreamed about french toast and sandwiches. I was very active, and I was eating lots of protein-rich foods whenever I got hungry.

I did this religiously for two months and guess what happened. My weight did not change, not one pound. My body got stronger, and my muscles firmed up, but my weight stayed the same for two months. I was appalled and angry then, but now I understand. Although I was eliminating some of my body's need for excess fat by eating to satisfy my hunger signals, I was not eating a high quality diet. There was no variety! And because of the exercise, I was creating another physiological need for muscle fat as my musculature developed.

Apparently the two needs balanced out, and I did not lose or gain by the scale. I might have actually burned some fat away, but because muscle is more dense tissue and weighs more than fat, I made up for the fat loss in larger, weightier muscles. I truly resembled a well-conditioned wrestler, but I still weighed 155 lbs. I became even more desperate.

DIET/EXERCISE BINGE—EATING/SITTING BINGE

You see, fat and muscles go together. But, too much of both is too much! When I went off the Atkins Diet, and everybody does sooner or later, I also gave up the exercise. I had had it! I never did like running that much. This pattern is typical: diet/exercise binging followed by eating/sitting binges. Remarkably, as I went back to more normal foods and stopped trying so hard, accepting my natural activity level, I began to lose weight! The weight loss didn't last, however, because I didn't really understand what to do to keep it off.

Medically speaking, muscles atrophy or deteriorate with disuse, just as they build up with use. The newly bedridden patient gradually begins to lose weight. If his diet is adequate, part of this loss represents muscle loss.

This is a normal physiological phenomenon, just as my weight gain with vigorous exercise and a high-protein diet was a normal adaptation. If you remember the principles behind these changes, you'll better understand your own body, your weight problem, and getting slim.

CHAPTER 4
OVEREATING:
SORTING OUT THE CAUSES

WHERE AND HOW YOU EAT

Where you choose to eat is different from what and when you eat. Wouldn't it be nice if you could eat anywhere at all and still be thin? You can! Almost every morning I gather stray dishes from various rooms in the house to be washed in the kitchen. Except for an evening meal in the dining room, my family seems to get hungry everywhere but the eating area! It's inconvenient, gathering the plates and glasses from everywhere, but we all enjoy eating in different places, sometimes while we do different things.

IT DOESN'T MATTER

Where you eat does not have an effect on your weight. In spite of the many diet manuals which say you must be sitting down to eat, or you must not have the television on, or you must be in the kitchen, these things don't matter. Naturally thin people don't think about such things. There is nothing magically nonfattening about sitting down at the table to eat, nor is there anything fattening about eating in front of the TV. Even midnight eating in bed has no appreciable effect on how fat or thin you are. You can eat wherever you want to and feel most comfortable at a given moment. The places might change with your moods and appetites. That's OK as long as you are eating real food to satisfy your real hunger.

THE "50-CHEWS-THEN-SWALLOW" DELUSION

Speed eating has a bad name, too, from what the old diet books say. But fast eating can be fun and natural, especially when you're hungry and in a hurry! Eating slowly, lingering over a special culinary creation is just as nice at a different time, a different place. Let yourself go the way your body feels like going—fast and furious, slow and serious, or anywhere in between. The speed at which you eat does not affect your weight significantly, either, so please, don't count your bites before they're swallowed. Just eat the way you feel like eating and enjoy it for a change.

THE LITTLE PLATE TRICK

The little plate trick never tricked my appetite. For those unfamiliar with the incredible lengths to which people will go to try to get around their bodies' hunger, I'll explain. There's a theory out (it's usually hooked up to the "count-fifty-chews-before-swallowing" idea), that the larger the plate you use, the smaller your portion of food seems. The proponents of this theory suggest that the dieter only use the smaller salad or luncheon plate so the portion they serve themselves will look proportionately larger than the same amount of food on a dinner plate.

To me this is ludicrous. Use a serving platter, if the mood strikes you. As long as you are in touch with your body's fuel-need signals, you'll stop when you're full anyway. And you'll have saved an extra dish!

Eat, Drink and Be Merry: You'll Never Diet Again

Finally, eating and drinking go together. Do not try to artificially separate them because some crazy diet manual said that drinks and stir-fry shouldn't get mixed up down there. It is most natural to drink beverages during a meal, especially during a salty meal. Don't fight it. And don't worry about it, either.

OVEREATING AND OVERWEIGHT: OTHER INFLUENCES

The rest of this chapter covers five other important factors which influence eating and overeating behavior: heredity, gender, emotions, extreme obesity, and cycle resistance.

HEREDITY VS. ENVIRONMENT

NONINHERITED (ENVIRONMENTAL) INFLUENCES ON BODY WEIGHT

Nongenetic factors cover over 99% of all cases of obesity, so if you've been blaming the genes, consider these things carefully.

1. Ignoring and suppressing the body's fuel-need signals is a learned behavior. It is completely unnatural and leads to the adaptive maintenance of excess weight. Learned behaviors and attitudes are not inherited.
2. Fat children tend to come from fat parents, not because they inherit the fat (more often than not, very obese mothers have normal-weight

infants and children), but because these parents inadvertently teach their children unhealthy eating habits. They also artificially control their eating according to their fears and misinformation.

3. Obese parents who allow their children to own their own diets have normally lean children. As these children grow up, they, too, may develop obesity, but it is not inherited. It is most likely a combination of ignorance, fear, misinformation, and the consequent cycle of undereating and overeating.

INHERITED TRAITS WHICH AFFECT BODY WEIGHT

Of course, there are certain aspects of the shape and quality of the human body which are determined, at least in part, by heredity, including the tendency to gain weight easily. Environment also has its impact on these traits.

First, the body type is inherited from parents. This includes height, bone size, distribution of normal fat, tendencies for distribution of abnormal fat, basic muscle mass, proportion, posture, and gait.

Second, a person's physiological sensitivities and strengths (resistance) can be inherited. This is where a predisposition to obesity lies. Some bodies can tolerate hunger and delayed eating better than others, and these are probably inherited traits. They don't overreact to food deprivation and go right to work on storing food. The body which is sensitive to the availability of food stores fat more readily in response to famine situations.

Third, we inherit tendencies toward certain physical and physiological diseases. Physical coordination has inherent properties. Metabolic rate is subject to hereditary influences. Food-taste preferences may be shared by parents and their children, partly because of shared genes. We also inherit all aspects of appearance, including coloring, shape, size, and flexibility of body parts, skin and hair.

PREDISPOSITION IS NOT CAUSE

Although we have no control over our heredity, predispositions or sensitivities that we inherit are not causes. We do have control over many of the environmental factors which combine with our predispositions to cause problems. We can change the availability of food in our environment by choosing to buy and eat food differently.

GENDER

CHANGES AT PUBERTY

I have been asked why in certain families women seem to be the only ones afflicted with weight problems. Actually, it has much less to do with family than gender.

SLIM ADOLESCENT BOYS: HOW DO THEY DO IT?

Boys go through puberty at about the same time as girls, and it is usually a stressful and difficult period of adjustment for them as well as girls. But, boys rarely develop weight problems during adolescence while it is common in girls. If teenage boys do have a problem with fat, it is that they seem to have too little of it. That is certainly not because they don't eat enough food. Active, adolescent boys are famous for their enormous appetites and their lean, muscular bodies. Are they just the favored few? How do their bodies manage all those double cheeseburgers and french fries? In a way, adoles-

cent boys are perfect examples of the fact that eating a
lot of food, by itself, doesn't cause obesity!

THE DIFFERENCE

There are other factors to consider here. Men have
higher metabolic rates. They burn more fuel in general
than women do. Also, men are proportionately more
muscular than women (women have a relatively larger
proportion of fat), which adds to the already greater
energy requirements of the male body. In general, men
are just bigger than women, and heavier, using more
energy for comparable amounts of activity because of
this weight difference.

These are three important reasons why men generally
can and do eat more food than women. Their appetites
and capacities for food are naturally greater in relation
to their bodies' greater fuel demands. This appetite/
need relationship is dependent on the diet ownership
of the men and women being compared. But none of
these things completely explains why women seem to be
more often plagued by obesity than their brothers and
husbands. What's the key to this part of the feminine
mystique?

GIRLS! WHAT'S GOING ON?

Earlier in the book I talked about the menarche, the
beginning of the menstrual period in women. This
event is brought on by female hormones which are controlled by the pituitary gland in the brain of the developing young girl. These hormones have many physiological and psychological effects, one of which is the
deposit of new fatty tissue on the body.

In order to deposit new fat, the body requires extra
fuel intake to handle the girls energy and metabolic
requirements. Her body signals the need for this additional fuel by increasing her appetite and possibly

changing her tastes slightly toward richer, more fat-producing foods. The overall effect is an increase in fuel intake, both quantitatively and qualitatively.

These changes occur gradually, without the slightest effort on the part of the young woman. Her body naturally develops into the childbearing stage quite apart from her own ideas of when and how these things should happen.

If the young woman stays out of her body's way and is allowed to own her own diet with plenty of real foods, she will remain slim as she was during her childhood, except for a subtle softening of her body's angles. But if she becomes anxious about her changing appetite and developing body and struggles against her increased appetite, she will forfeit ownership of her diet and start the Feast-or-Famine Cycle with her first dieting efforts.

This most often happens when the girl has an obese mother who is a dieter. Because the girl, like her mother, erroneously associates hunger and eating with obesity, she is prone to fear and resist her appetite while her brother, unafraid, eats with abandon. She grows plump in her fear, and her brother cannot seem to eat enough to keep up with his body's demands.

TEENAGE DIETING: SERIOUS PROGNOSIS

Once the Feast-or-Famine Cycle is firmly established in the adolescent girl, she is likely to gain more weight than she can diet off. She may manage limited control of her weight gain, but her dieting will inadvertently create the need for extra fat. The pattern is self-defeating. Her body needs the excess fat stores to survive the famine diets she imposes on it, so the harder she tries to lose weight, the more she will need to stay fat. She is fat because she tries so hard to get slim. Her brother, on the other hand, enjoys a slim, muscular body because he is not trying at all. He is eating!

Have you ever heard a fat person say, "The harder I try, the fatter I get!"? How true it is!

In order to become slim naturally and permanently, the obese person must begin to eat more like the adolescent boy—fearlessly. These young men don't think about calories or nutrition or when or how much they ate at the last meal. They sometimes eat huge amounts of real food when they are hungry and they always eat until they are completely satisfied. That's why they are slim. Their bodies do not need excessive, burdensome fat because they are continually supplying their bodies' fuel needs according to their hunger, and nothing but their hunger.

THE MENSTRUAL CYCLE

I am not implying that female hormones, by themselves, produce the tendency for obesity. But I believe that the menstrual cycle does predispose women to the vicious Feast-or-Famine Cycle. Because the menstrual cycle is a natural body rhythm which affects appetite and eating behavior, the normal cyclical changes that occur are easily exaggerated in the body of the woman who thinks she must control her weight by traditional dieting. Instead of eating a little more or less real food as her body's signals change, the dieter fights the urge to eat and ends up overeating or undereating most of the time.

ANYBODY CAN BE NATURALLY THIN

Although men are also vulnerable to the Feast-or-Famine Cycle (see Ch.7), they do not have such a built-in ebb and flow of appetite to start the Cycle and keep it going. Women probably have a greater challenge to trust their bodies because of this monthly cycle and their slower metabolisms, but everyone has a chance to be free from the ups and downs of traditional dieting. It will probably take a woman longer to lose the extra fat she has acquired by dieting off and on, but her thin figure will be just as permanent and easy to maintain as a man's.

EMOTIONAL OVEREATING

Primary overeating, like primary or essential hypertension, from which I borrowed the term, does not exist. Primary overeating (overeating in and of itself without an underlying physical cause) never occurs. There is always a reason for overeating or people wouldn't do it. The causative factor is almost always physical. The emotional side has been blamed much more often than it deserves. Diet literature often purports that people most commonly overeat because of stress and emotional problems. This is not true. So if you have labeled yourself an emotional or spiritual jellyfish, take heart. There are other more concrete, normal reasons.

"EMOTIONAL EATING" IS REALLY PHYSICAL

These normal reasons are right in your body, not your mind. They are physical and they make good sense once you become aware of them. People who are fat often have emotional problems, but that is because they are human. The problems didn't make them overeat and get fat, their bodies did. Oh, they all helped their poor bodies along by going hungry trying in the traditional route to lose weight, but their bodies did the overwhelming bulk of the work. I'll explain.

THE ADAPTIVE RESPONSE TO STRESS IS NOT HUNGER

The body's normal, adaptive response to stress is to avoid food. Remember the fight/flight illustration at the beginning of the book? What is the body's basic physiological response to external stress?

Suppose a vicious dog suddenly dashes out of the bushes, right into the path of a lanky young letter carrier. How will his stomach react? It will become queasy. When a threat presents itself to the normal, thin body, the body prepares automatically to fight or flee. The digestive tract shuts down, allowing the blood to circulate where it's needed most—in the muscles for action and the brain for clear, fast thinking. Decisions have to be made instantly and the body must be prepared to act according to those decisions. This is no time to digest lunch!

A SATISFIED APPETITE SHUTS DOWN WITH STRESS

So in the normal, lean body, the appetite is physiologically suppressed under stressful conditions. This is also true of psychological stressors. The very thought of an upcoming performance or speech will stop the gastric juices fast while the heart skips a beat and a lump in the throat forces a dry swallow. This elimination of normal appetite under stress is transient and adaptive, promoting the body's survival.

What about fat people? They often have the opposite reaction when something stressful happens. Why?

WHY EATING IS A STRESS RELIEVER TO DIETERS

Fat people are hungry people. They almost always suffer from an exaggerated, undersatisfied hunger because of their chronic attempts to ignore their appetites. Chronically hungry overweight people don't experience hunger suppression under stress because of their exaggerated need for food. This need is physical, not emotional.

When there has been a famine (as there always has in the obese person) and the body has been forced to tolerate hunger, stress plus the availability of food produce a paradoxical effect. Instead of representing an additional stress to the already stress-challenged body, food becomes a stress relief to the hungry fat person. Given a choice, the body will naturally relieve as many stresses as possible, eliminating those stresses over which it has some control. Many stressors that the body encounters are unrelievable, like the three-minute speech which is not actually due for several days. The body must cope with the anxiety of anticipation, and until the speech is given, the anxiety is unrelievable stress.

Let's say that the person who is to give the speech is overweight. She is usually trying to diet or control her appetite, however unsuccessfully, but things like this little talk in front of an audience really make dieting impossible. In fact, stresses most often trigger terrible binges and depression. Why?

OVERWEIGHT DIETERS USUALLY EAT UNDER STRESS

The stress of chronic and excessive hunger is relievable. The body can eliminate the discomfort of such hunger by causing the person to eat, usually far in excess of her immediate needs. Her body's need to store and replace fat causes overeating. This is exactly what happens to the obese person who is faced with an unrelievable stress plus chronic undersatisfied hunger. The body fixes the hunger and copes with the rest. As long as the person is on the Feast or Famine Cycle, she will likely overeat when under stress. Once the Cycle is broken, however, even while she is overweight, her normal food-avoidance response will work in the presence of other stressors. Yours will, too. Just let it happen.

In summary, emotional and physical stress, without the ongoing presence of undersatisfied hunger, does not normally cause overeating. Stress normally causes eating-avoidance, which most naturally thin people experience. Obese people experience the opposite effect. They tend to overeat under stressful conditions because food represents a stress-relief to the body. Instead of the normal additive stress effect that it has on the hunger-satisfied thin, food offers irresitable relief to the overhungry.

THE EMOTIONS THAT CAUSE OVEREATING

There is one emotion which has a universal effect on the eating behavior of overweight people. This emotion is often the most powerful force in keeping the Feast-or-Famine Cycle going. It indirectly brings about overeating because it directly causes undereating and eating avoidance. This emotion is fear.

Fear and anxiety propel the vicious Feast-or-Famine Cycle. Fear keeps the hunger signals quiet. Fear of what? Fear of eating. People who have been trying to lose weight by dieting are convinced that eating makes them and keeps them fat. They are afraid of food and afraid to eat. They are anxious about eating almost all the time, whether dieting or not.

Overcoming this fear is no easy task. It is almost a phobia with some veteran dieters. These people have the greatest obstacle to deal with in becoming slim. They must replace their fear with faith. Because of their new understanding, they must stop feeling afraid to eat and start believing in their bodies. Once they begin to act on their faith and understanding, their emotions will follow.

OTHER EMOTIONS THAT INFLUENCE THE FEAST-OR-FAMINE CYCLE

Certain emotions are especially powerful in fueling the Feast-or-Famine Cycle. We know that they do not directly cause overeating and weight gain because these things are controlled by the body in response to undereating. But, besides fear, do emotions cause famines? Yes! Two emotions have a lot to do with dieting and eating-avoidance.

EMOTIONS THAT CAUSE FAMINES

Dieting or going without food when you're hungry is painful. This pain can be used as a form of self-punishment for people who feel guilty or ashamed. And what do overweight people feel guilty about? Their overeating, of course, not to mention all the "bad" things they choose to eat. And what do overweight people feel ashamed about? Their bodies, of course, and their inability to control their eating or lose weight, which everyone everywhere has always said they should be able to do with a little willpower.

So, shame and guilt cause famines whenever a person tries to pay for her "sins" by the self-inflicted pain of unsatisfied hunger. Dieting serves an important emotional need in this way; fat people feel better about themselves when they are dieting (in pain) because of these emotions. Dieting temporarily relieves feelings of shame and guilt and overeating promotes these feelings.

The cycle looks like this:

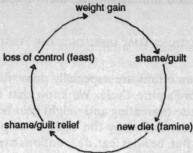

weight gain

loss of control (feast)

shame/guilt

shame/guilt relief

new diet (famine)

The Anti-Diet interrupts this cycle at two crucial points; the shame/guilt and the new diet fix. When a person learns that her weight gain is not a result of her laziness, apathy, lack of motivation or poor willpower, but rather a consequence of her determined but misguided efforts, the shame she feels diminishes instantly. She feels understood and begins to have compassion for herself for the first time. And as she begins to accept her hunger as normal and her eating as her right and responsibility (even while she is still obese!) the guilt diminishes too.

Relatively guilt and shame-free, she loses the urge to punish herself. And the diet fix, once she understands the Feast-or-Famine Cycle, is no longer a fix at all. The pain of going hungry serves no purpose and consequently, she avoids it. (Remember, it's adaptive to avoid pain.) The cycle is broken.

ADDICTION AND OBESITY

Obesity is not the result of a food or eating addiction. Everyone is addicted to food in the truest sense. That is, everyone (even the thinnest people) would suffer withdrawal symptoms if food were unavailable. Many individuals and organizations falsely label distorted eating behavior as an addiction. This is misleading and unhelpful in solving the basic problem which is undereating, not overeating. The food addiction approach actually does more harm than good, and in my experience has never led anyone to a lasting recovery. Alleged "food addicts" are taught and do believe that they must be on guard against food forever. What a trap.

EXTREME OBESITY AND THE ROLE OF STRESS

In the last section I explained that the body tries to eliminate any relievable stresses in its environment. It is prone to cope with the least number of stressors possible in a given situation. Very often an unrelievable stress provokes the body of the dieter to begin the feasting part of the Feast-or-Famine Cycle. Her body eliminates the stress of chronic undersatisfied hunger by causing her to overeat, leaving behind only the stressors over which it has no influence.

The failing dieter thinks that her willpower mysteriously broke down at a stressful moment, as it often does. Or she thinks she used the new stress as an excuse to satisfy her sick craving to overeat. These things are only partly true. It is really her body that coerced her into overeating. Her body's adaptive tendency is to eliminate any relievable stresses in the environment, leaving only the unrelievable ones to cope with by other means.

STRESS: THE OVEREATING TRIGGER

Since food represents a stress relief to the chronic diet-conscious person, she most often eats when she is under stress. Her body overrules her misguided willpower, and she reluctantly (and often ashamedly) overeats to make up for her most recent attempt to lose weight. But the most interesting and tragic part of this stress/overeating cycle is yet to be exposed.

OVEREATING RELIEVES CHRONIC HUNGER

The Feast-or-Famine Cycle starts in the slightly overweight person when she attempts to lose weight by traditional methods. Misguided, she imposes an artificial season of famine on her body, beginning the Cycle with undersatisfied hunger. As life's normal stressful moments come, this new dieter encounters stresses in her hungry, first-diet life. And because her body can eliminate the hunger of her reduction diet (and also the stress of that hunger) by eating and overeating, that's exactly what she does. When she gets tense or upset, she overeats, beyond her current appetite and beyond her understanding.

UNDEREATING RELIEVES GUILT AND FEAR

During the intermittent famines (diets or controlled eating) that follow, she loses weight because her body will adapt temporarily to an environment of lowered food availability and forfeit some of its fat in order to survive. But she regains that fat, and often more, once the feasting begins. In time, she gradually gains weight. The more she diets, the fatter she gets.

OBESITY BECOMES THE CHRONIC STRESS

At some point, her obesity becomes the unrelievable stress that causes overeating, and the Cycle propels itself. The very fatness of her body and the desperation she feels at not being able to diet successfully begin to trigger the feasting part of the Cycle. So great is the internal conflict, self-hatred, rejection, and pain that other stressors become relatively insignificant. Ironically, the hunger goes on and on and on.

Hopelessly Overweight

Eventually, very obese, she seems to give up altogether in order to survive emotionally. And that's the best word for it—survival. There is so little joy, so little love, so little understanding. In place of these things there is an unbelievable amount of suffering. If you are or have ever been very obese, you know. If you have ever had any type of weight problem, you can imagine. If you have always eaten freely and never had to think twice about your weight, you cannot imagine the pain.

Token Attempts to Diet Keep the Cycle Going

Oh, she may make some token attempts to diet. Often they are extreme, unhealthy, and short-lived. These efforts are perhaps more for the sake of other people or to maintain a semblance of determination, than for the obese person herself. She is truly without hope. Ironically, her dieting efforts to save face keep her locked in the vicious Cycle of overeating and starving and needing fat, all for the sake of her pitiful survival.

Revise Your Attitudes

When you see a fat person, I hope your new understanding of her plight will make you far more compassionate. She is not fat because of sin. She is not weak willed or given to an unnatural lust for food. She is not lazy or hung up or just naturally gross. She is not fat because of an emotional handicap, but she is severely emotionally handicapped because she is fat. She does not need the latest promise-laden quick-loss fad diet. She needs to learn about her body and what she can do to help it work the way it was intended to work.

Saints and Sinners

If you know someone who is extremely obese yet nice,

she is something of a saint. If you know a very fat person who is not nice, perhaps you can now understand part of the reason why. Neither of these people are likely to covet your pity, and it is not your sympathy that they need. They need information—true information for a change. Loan them this book. They will understand it better than anyone.

CYCLE RESISTANCE: NATURAL THINS

Many people do not realize what their bodies are like in their most adapted, lean condition, but some people do. They always have. They are naturally thin, and they usually don't know how lucky they are. They are often considered too thin, but they are almost always just right. They even have fat, just like heavier people, but their fat is easily camouflaged, hiding everywhere—in the muscles, around the internal organs, deep in the abdomen, and just under the skin. They need the amounts of fat they keep for smooth physiological functioning, not for surviving famines. The amount of this fat varies slightly within a normal range with seasonal climate changes, changes in the eating environment (vacations, holidays), changes in physiological need (activity level, pregnancy), and other stresses. These natural thins sometimes lose weight or gain a little, but as they keep ownership of their diets, they remain generally lean.

Naturally thin people seem to have been immunized against obesity. They just stay thin, no matter what they eat. They even get excessively hungry sometimes, but they don't go crazy and binge for two days. The Feast-or-Famine Cycle cannot seem to catch them. Why?

OBESITY VACCINE

In the section on heredity a few pages back I talked about inherited sensitivities and predispositions to obesity. Just as the fat-prone person is sensitive to the physiological effects of careless eating or famine diets, the natural thin inherently resists these effects. Their bodies are not so "tuned in to the environment". The obese-prone are actually better adapted because their bodies' sensitivities to food shortage are better suited to keeping them alive in a real environmental famine. But since real famines are unlikely in our culture, the natural thins do just fine. Those of us with sensitive but outdated adaptive responses have struggled endlessly. The end is finally in sight.

WEIGHT FLUCTUATIONS IN NATURAL THINS

Natural thins may nevertheless become vulnerable to weight gain at certain stages of life. If during these times they forfeit ownership of their diets and go on a typical reduction diet, they are in trouble. You know why. They will begin the Feast-or-Famine Cycle and, because of the artificial lack of food during the famines, their bodies will develop a need for excess fat, and they will continue to gain weight off and on. This explains why people who once enjoyed a slim, effortlessly lean figure get fat "all of a sudden". Actually, it doesn't happen all of a sudden. It takes time. They just realize it all of a sudden.

TOO THIN

At the other end of the spectrum, some people are genuinely too thin. Their thinness is not normal or adaptive. Either they have a disease like hyperthyroidism or, for some reason, they do not eat enough quality food. One way or another, their bodies are not running efficiently either.

Although there are slight differences in different groups' adaptive fat requirements, these differences are so small that they are not usually noticeable. The most adaptive condition for any body, even a pregnant one, is nonobese. And underweight is no more adaptive than fat.

EATING DISORDERS

ANOREXIA NERVOSA

One very serious mental illness which involves dangerous underweight is Anorexia Nervosa. The main symptoms of this illness are compulsive self-starvation, body weight significantly below normal limits, preoccupation with food and eating, and a severely distorted body image. People with Anorexia Nervosa get off the Feast-or-Famine Cycle on the Famine side, and they have to lose touch with reality to do it. This disease can be fatal, leading to heart or kidney failure.

If you have any of these symptoms (or other people say you do), or you know anyone who does, contact a professional in mental health or medicine, preferably a psychiatrist.

BULEMIA NERVOSA

Another eating disorder which has, according to some, reached epidemic proportions in the past decade, is bulemia. People with this disease have food binges and then force themselves to throw up afterward, in order to control weight gain. The binge-purge cycle may occur many times a day. Bulemics also become preoccupied with eating and food, often abuse laxatives, and invariably have a distorted body image.

I have never met a bulemic who wasn't on the Feast-or-Famine Cycle. Every bulemic I have interviewed or coached was, along with binging and purging, trying to eat less or not eating in an effort to lose weight. There's no such thing as a Feast without a Famine! Mysteriously, when these women learn to eat enough real food on a daily basis according to their hunger signals, their binging disappears. And without binges and fear of weight gain that go with them, they no longer need to purge or throw up. So they don't. So much for the food addiction theory.

There are also psychological factors to consider in some cases of bulemia, but the first approach to recovery must be understanding the Feast-or-Famine Cycle. That's where the binging begins—at the famine stage. Eliminate the famines (diets) and most often that's the end of compulsive overeating and vomiting.

In cases where an individual cannot eat freely according to her hunger signals in spite of her understanding of the Cycle, because of fear or other emotional issues, I advise her to seek professional counsel. There are many therapists who deal with eating disorders now. However, no matter how much therapy she receives, unless she deals with her fear of eating and obesity and gives up her efforts to control her weight by dieting, the Cycle cannot be broken and her pain and symptoms will continue.

CHAPTER 5
FOOD AND PREJUDICE

GIMMICK DIETS PROMOTE SENSELESS FOOD PREJUDICES

DR. ATKIN'S RESEARCH:
GIVING CARBOHYDRATES A BAD NAME

Dr. Atkins discovered that, in the absence of a significant amount of carbohydrate in the diet, the body will use the next most combustible source of fuel available. In his low-carbohydrate, high-protein, high-fat diet, that source is protein. Protein supplies the body with ready fuel for energy and metabolic needs. Dietary fat is not usable without adequate carbohydrates. In the absence of adequate dietary protein and any usable form of dietary fat, the body metabolizes its own stored fat to meet its remaining fuel needs.

I have already alluded to my experience with the Atkins diet. Actually, this diet does cause weight loss for many obese people who follow it well. Dr. Atkins had two very good suggestions in his diet: You can eat whenever you get hungry, and you can eat until you are completely satisfied. But his whole theory is based on what he considered the necessary elimination of dietary carbohydrates. For his system to work, carbohydrate foods must be eliminated or severely restricted. Otherwise all the fat consumed can be used by the body.

But your body *needs* carbohydrates, whether you are as fat as a bass fiddle or as skinny as a fiddle's bow. Carbohydrates serve many vital roles in your body's metabolic and physiological processes. To eliminate them from your diet artificially puts tremendous unnecessary stress on your body. If you are eating lots of protein and fat, the hunger of eat-less dieting may be eliminated, but there is another kind of hunger to take its place— chronic carbohydrate hunger.

There is absolutely nothing the matter with carbohydrates. Dr. Atkins simply thought that, because of the role carbohydrates play in dietary fat metabolism, they were the most logical food group to eliminate. After all, who comprises the largest group of consumers of carbohydrate-rich foods? Fat people. The evidence abounds! So does the prejudice.

The problem with Dr. Atkins's Diet is that it is a famine diet. It is not a food-quantity famine. It is a food-quality famine. Man cannot live by bread alone, but neither was man intended to live without bread at all! If you have ever tried the Atkins diet, you have probably experienced your body's revulsion against protein and its craving for carbohydrates.

Carbohydrates do not make people fat. What does? Eating too much? Stress? Foods with too much fat? Emotions? I hope your answers are no, no, no, and no. Food, eating, and feelings do not make people fat. Famines make people fat.

I was at the grocery store once when all the shelves had just been stocked. I was awestruck by the incredible abundance all around me and sobered by the many overweight shoppers anxiously selecting dietetic foods. I wanted so much to tell each one the key.

Traditional dieting must change if we are to halt the

problem of obesity in the world. Dr. Atkins was right about a lot of things. You can eat when you are hungry until you are completely full, and you can still lose weight. I say you not only can but *must.* I also change the no-carbohydrates policy to "all this and carbohydrates too!"

FAST AND TEMPORARY VS. SLOW AND PERMANENT

You will not lose weight quickly when you break the Feast-or-Famine Cycle. You will probably gain weight at first, then level off and gradually begin to drop extra pounds. Dr. Atkins offered quick loss without hunger, but he did not offer permanent weight control because his diet regimen is too difficult and unnatural to stay on. To achieve permanent weight loss you have to trade the time it takes to get thin for a lifetime of slimness. You must wait and learn how your body can become slim without your interference. It does take longer, but it is forever. And it doesn't hurt.

THE BREAD AND POTATO PHOBIA

A phobia is an unrealistic fear. Dieters are deathly afraid of bread, potatoes, and other perfectly harmless real foods, like pasta. They are afraid because they think (they have been told!) that bread and potatoes make people fat. This is not true. I trust that by now I don't need to explain why. If you doubt my word, go back and start reading the book over again. You are suffering from an advanced case of dietitis, I'm sure. Do not be alarmed, though. The phobias, paranoid thought patterns, and other troublesome symptoms will disappear as you arrest the disease.

One suggestion: There is a clinically tested psychological trick that may help you. Try buying and eventually eating the objects of your exaggerated fear. I know this is frightening at first. Try as you may, you probably can't imagine being strong enough to do such a courageous thing. But I do believe that in time you will be able to actually enjoy, yes, enjoy these frightening foods. Good luck!

HAVING IT YOUR WAY

Eggs are a good example of a terrific real food. If you like them, your body can use eggs well for fuel and nutrition. When you do eat eggs, cook or order them the way you like them best. Maybe you'll change from time to time. Some days you may want poached on toast. Other times scrambled may sound better. Do not have your eggs poached or boiled if you don't like them that way. You'll feel cheated.

You must not cheat your hunger, appetite, or taste buds while you're losing weight. These needs were not meant to be ignored. But they can be important guidelines in selecting a balanced and nutritious diet.

If you do like poached eggs, get them that way. Don't order them fried in bacon grease just to defy the old diet restrictions. If you don't prefer the extra fat, your body doesn't need it anymore. Be honest. Have all foods prepared the way you like them most at the moment, and stay open to change as your need for fat diminishes. Your taste for fat and fat-producing foods will diminish with your body's changing needs.

CRAVINGS AND ADDICTIONS

Everyone is addicted to food in the truest sense of the word. We would all suffer serious withdrawal effects, ultimately leading to death, if food were eliminated from the environment. No one, however spiritual, can get along without it, and obviously those who try to do so, in a limited sense, suffer the consequences of the traditional approach to weight loss: obesity, malnutrition, blood-sugar imbalances, blood-vessel fat problems, dry skin, dermatitis, bowel and digestive disturbances, nervousness, depression, and a wide assortment of other physical, emotional, psychological, social, and spiritual maleffects. There is probably no limit to the list.

COMMON HOUSEHOLD DRUGS

Caffeine, nicotine, and alcohol are all drugs. Like the vast majority of drugs that humans have learned to use, they are basically good and useful drugs. But like antibiotics, these drugs can also be harmful when abused or overused, and the body suffers negative effects from the misuse of these basically good things.

The drugs themselves are not to blame for these ill effects in the same way that food is not the real culprit in diet failure. Food, coffee, wine, tobacco, and all such substances are simply available to us. We are the ones guilty of abuse. Sometimes we are guilty because of our ignorance, like the person caught in the Feast-or-Famine Cycle. But often we are guilty of drug abuse in full knowledge of what we are doing. We know that it is abuse because our bodies complain with symptoms of overload.

DRUG ABUSE IS COMMON

Many, many people use drugs inappropriately when they are hungry. Because we have been taught that eating too much causes us to get fat, we avoid eating. But the drive to eat when hunger strikes is so strong that, if we are bent on not eating, our bodies will opt for some kind of substitute to pacify our craving. The smoker has a cigarette, the homemaker has another cup of coffee, and toward evening, many people have a drink. These people are using drugs as food substitutes. This is not only maladaptive, it ultimately leads to the very thing they are all trying to fix: obesity.

There is no good earthly substitute for food. Drugs are very poor substitutes. Actually, the alcoholic beverage is the least of the three evils because at least it has some calories (admittedly, very poor quality calories) while cigarettes, coffee, or diet colas provide no nutritional substance whatever. Coffee with cream and sugar, yes, but we all know that traditional diets never, never allow a hungry, fat dieter the luxury of "fattening" cream and/or sugar in her coffee! Unfortunately, the positive aspect of the alcoholic beverage is cancelled out by the fact that it is a depressant. But then, this may have one positive side effect because the person may be more inclined to eat after the drink, which she should have done in the first place.

SPEEDING ON EMPTY

What about the stimulant effects of the other two—caffeine and nicotine? They do pep you up when you feel tired and hungry, and that effect temporarily makes you less compelled to eat. However, the pep effect without food has disastrous long-term effects. It increases the severity of your body's famine.

When you get hungry, your blood sugar is on the low side of normal. That is one of the ways your body senses its fuel need. So when you are hungry, your body needs fuel in the form of real foods that it can use well. When you, because you are dieting, avoid food and substitute a stimulant (coffee, a cigarette, any substance containing caffeine or nicotine, tanin in tea, amphetamines, or over-the-counter appetite suppressants) your body moves artificially into high gear without providing the necessary additional energy nutrients it needs to run at a faster pace. Not only is there a famine in the land by virtue of your reduction diet and anti-eating approach, there is an increased metabolic fuel demand.

Your body is not only forced to burn its glycogen and other fuel reserves under great physical duress, it must cope with the additional stress of keeping your blood sugar within the narrow safety limits without any ready fuel. It must burn the most readily available form of tissue as fast as possible to meet these extreme energy demands. Under such pressure, what does your body use for fuel? When it's out of glycogen stores, it uses muscle.

CANNIBALISM

In the absence of food, the next best source of ready fuel is internal protein. The protein stored in your body is in your muscles. So your body is forced by the high metabolism famine described above, to eat its own muscle tissue to keep up with the needs you impose on it. So, when you are dieting and you smoke, drink coffee or cola or tea, or take diet pills, your body is sometimes using its internal stores of protein (muscle), not fat, to meet your heightened energy and fuel needs. It's no wonder that a strict low-calorie regimen with lots of "free" beverages like black coffee, clear tea, and diet colas leaves the dieter weak, shaky, irritable, depressed and more vulnerable to disease.

BLOOD SUGAR

Disorders related to blood-sugar levels have become very common recently. That's understandable, too, with so many people going around trying not to eat when their bodies need food! What exactly is blood sugar and why is it getting to be such a problem?

DIABETES AND HYPOGLYCEMIA

"Blood sugar" is a medical term which refers to the level of ready energy fuel, glucose, circulating in the bloodstream. Another word for glucose is sugar. The blood-sugar level of an individual is constantly changing, like her blood pressure, but these changes normally occur within a range of safety. There is an upper and a lower limit of safety, but these limits are general and serve only as guidelines for diagnosis and treatment of disease.

If a person's blood-sugar level rises significantly above these normal limits and persists above the normal range, the body will eventually show symptoms of disease. Something is wrong in the body's ability to keep the blood sugar within healthy limits. This is the key symptom of diabetes—elevated blood sugar.

If the blood sugar falls below normal limits, other symptoms may signal problems in keeping the blood-sugar level high enough. This problem is generally referred to as hypoglycemia or low blood sugar.

If you have any questions about diabetes or hypoglycemia, ask your doctor.

Low blood sugar has become a household word. Almost everyone has heard the term used, and a significant number of people have been diagnosed as having the malady, but few people know what low blood sugar is and how it feels, even if they've had it. Common symptoms include irritability, short temper, anger, tension, rage, weakness, dizziness, nausea, headache, nervousness, sweating, crying, over-reaction, fear, panic, anxiety, extreme hunger, dry mouth, and blurred vision. Extreme low blood sugar can cause fainting, unconsciousness, or coma, and it can even lead to death.

A more common picture of low blood sugar is described earlier in the book. It's the first example of a chronic dieter. Another typical case of low blood sugar can be found on the freeway during rush-hour traffic. This victim is a gentleman with an empty stomach due to watching his weight (undereating). He skipped lunch. When I say gentleman, I use the term loosely because the person with low blood sugar, a lot of stress, and no food in sight is anything but gentle!

EMERGENCY FUEL SYSTEMS

Dieters who are running their bodies on an empty fuel tank are running on their bodies' emergency fuel systems (the body's mechanisms for producing more sugar when no source is available from food). Because the level of sugar circulating in the bloodstream is vital to the person's survival, her emergency systems try to keep that level within its critical limits—high enough, in the case of the dieter going hungry.

It is not simple, either. In fact, an active body and mind without ready fuel has to withstand considerable internal stress just to maintain. And the limits to which the body will go in order to stay alive under stress without food are phenomenal.

LOW-BLOOD-SUGAR ANTIDOTE

Persons who get symptoms of hypoglycemia need to protect their bodies from this metabolic energy crisis. They need to eat real foods whenever they get hungry until they are completely satisfied. They do not need to eat in advance of their hunger, but they must eat as immediately as possible when they begin to feel hungry. They must never wait too long. They have to prevent their blood sugar from dropping too low. It is important for these people, especially, to carry emergency food with them.

Perfect emergency foods are combinations of carbohydrates, protein, and fat because each type of food fuel is broken down by the body at a different rate. Carbohydrates can be digested quickly for an immediate blood-sugar boost. Proteins are slower burning and have a less-dramatic effect but are longer acting in keeping the blood sugar stable. Fats burn still more slowly and stay with you over a longer time.

So, if you have experienced some of the signs of low blood sugar described here, and most people have, keep portable, quality real food on hand when you're away from home—in the car, in your purse, in a desk drawer at the office, wherever hunger might strike unexpectedly.

If you use this food supply to help your body keep your blood sugar level stable, you will feel better. You will have more energy and patience. Your moods will be more stable and positive. Your body will be more relaxed because it won't have internal "emergencies" to cope with every day. There are enough real emergencies for your body to withstand. Don't add blood-sugar crises to the list.

CRAVINGS ARE NEED SIGNALS

SUGAR BABIES: UNDERSTANDING THE "SWEET TOOTH"

Babies and little children love sugar and almost all sweet foods. They have a natural preference for sweet things. The original sweet food is mother's breast milk, of course. It is sweet and dilute, having proportionately more sugar and water than other types of milk. Why doesn't breast milk have more protein instead? Isn't protein the most important nutrient for a fast-growing baby? No, more sugar and water is better for babies. That's why it's there, and that's why they like it. Just what is it about sugar that babies like and apparently need?

First, sugar is the simplest form of food to use for energy, requiring the least amount of energy to digest. Therefore, it burns completely and efficiently with little stress to a baby's sensitive digestive tract.

Second, any sugar eaten in excess of the baby's fuel requirements is readily converted into fat and stored for future use. I will discuss the importance of fat for a baby after the newborn stage in Ch. 7.

Interestingly, even babies from the most obese mothers do not come out of the womb fat. It would be maladaptive, causing a tighter squeeze through the birth canal. But once the baby begins to get milk from the breast, a few days postpartum, it begins to eat more fuel than its little body is using up. The rest is stored in fat. This fat serves as insulation, padding, fuel during sleep when food is not available, and emergency fuel for illness.

Babies crave foods that taste sweet because their bodies need to use the efficient fuel sugar, and they need the fat that their bodies are able to manufacture from sugar.

What about fat people? They crave sweets, too, and junk foods. Don't their bodies need protein and real foods instead? No, frankly, they don't.

DIETERS CRAVE FOODS THEY NEED

Fat people need the foods they crave, just like babies do. They are fat because they have an exaggerated, maladaptive need for fat created by dieting or ignoring their hunger. Since the famines generally get more severe and/or longer in duration, over time the physiological need for fat grows greatly. As this need for fat increases, so does her craving for fat-producing foods: sugar, fat, sweet foods, fat foods, junk foods—lots of them.

When fat people are feasting after a famine, they appear not to care about their fatness at all. They seem to be eating without one conscience pang. But overweight people know how much they do care in spite of how they act. Only they know how desperately they have wanted to be thin. When their efforts mock them with more and more fat, they hide their desire and sometimes their eating, too. It is painful to be so big, so hungry, and so humiliated at the same time. They give in to their cravings with apparent abandon, eating the very foods they are "supposed to avoid." Yet these are the foods that their bodies *need* in order to survive. Their cravings and their needs go perfectly together, just like a baby and sweet breast milk.

ARROGANT THINS

Thin people often take pride in their thinness, even if they are overweight, though relatively thin. They take credit for the superior shape of their bodies, saying, "Thank you, I work at it!" What they mean to say is that it isn't easy for anybody, but at least they are not like the really fat people who never try at all. They share their latest diet tips with those "less disciplined," more to flaunt their self-control than to help. They have no understanding of the obese person's no-win dilemma.

The fact is, these prideful thins often have not tried as hard as their heavier counterparts. They are not as sensitive to the availability of food, and their bodies are not as efficient at adapting to famine diets by storing fat. We all need to understand and have compassion.

♣

SETPOINT: A COMMENT

The idea of setpoint is supposed to explain why dieters have such a hard time getting below a certain weight. Because of this established setpoint, the body purportedly protects itself from losing weight below a certain point which it sets arbitrarily. But it does not make sense to me that the body clings, without cause, to a certain amount of excess fat.

This is what this popular setpoint notion suggests. How depressing! This concept further implies that if you want to lose weight beyond the setpoint, you must change your setpoint somehow by fighting the body.

I agree that the body resists change and may fight the disequilibrium which results from quick-weight-loss program. That's why we often hear the comment, "I can starve myself and not lose a pound!"

But there is no mystery as to why the body protects the pounds that we consider unnecessary. They are necessary to the dieter's body. They ensure survival, the body's primary goal.

So I basically agree with the setpoint concept but I disagree that this fascinating mechanism for body-weight maintenance is either senseless or arbitrary. It is a mechanism for survival to be respected, not carelessly subdued.

Changing your body's setpoint starts with changing its need for fat, and you can only do that by changing when and what you eat.

FAMINE POINT

An understanding of this term will help you avoid eating too little as you begin to allow your body to adjust to an environment of optimum food availability. The famine point is the amount of food or quality of food *below* which your body will maintain and store fat. In

other words, each individual must eat at a certain balanced, caloric *minimum* in order to eliminate the need
for fat. We are not talking about upper limits here, we
are considering minimum standards for amount and
variety of foods to ensure permanent weight loss. What
happens if your eating isn't up to these standards? You
might lose weight, temporarily, but it will be famine
weight loss and you know what comes after a famine.

I will not tell you what these standards are because I
can't. They are different for everybody, and they differ
for one individual from day to day. How will you know?
Your body will tell you. How will your body tell you? Signals.

LISTEN CAREFULLY

Your body communicates its fuel needs via certain signals: appetite, hunger, cravings, satiation, and nausea. If
you have been on the Feast-or-Famine Cycle, you have
probably damaged your body's delicate communications system. Don't worry. Bodies are incredibly resil-
ient. They tend to forgive and forget once you begin to
treat them with the care and respect they deserve. What
about the famine point? Listen carefully to your body,
give it what it needs, and you will eat enough to lose
weight eventually.

CHAPTER 6
EATING ON TIME

BODY SIGNALS

The term, body language, refers to a physical communication system which aids, and sometimes contradicts, what you say. It includes gesture, posture, facial expression, and vocal resonance and pitch. Body signals do not involve communication between people (interpersonal) but rather communication within one person (innerpersonal). Specifically, it is the physical part of you "talking" to the mental part of you.

COMMUNICATION BREAKDOWN

Obviously, without your mind your body cannot literally speak. However, a communication system requires only a set of understandable symbols in order to be effective. We have already discussed some of these symbols (physical sensations) and their interpretations. Everyone's body has such a "language" and depends on it for survival. But, as I suggested in the last section, many dieters have experienced a communication breakdown with their bodies. Why does this breakdown occur? What happens between the Feast-or-Famine dieter and her body to damage this once-healthy communication system?

There are two main reasons for this communication gap. They are the same as those which cause interpersonal communication breakdowns.

MISTRUST

The first problem is mistrust. As we have discussed earlier, the depravation dieter does not trust her body, especially her hunger sensations. You know what happens when a person tries to ignore or deny her body's attempts to communicate its fuel needs. She eventually gets fat.

FAULTY LISTENING SKILLS

The second communication problem is not listening. The Feast-or-Famine dieter does not listen to what her body is trying to tell her. She works hard not to listen because listening is natural.

Unfortunately, poor listening skills always lead to the deterioration of a relationship. Instead of being a friend to her body, she becomes its archenemy, trying to outsmart its unreasonable whims. But these "whims" are just its natural need signals.

The ultimate result is a complete communication breakdown between a desperate dieter and her determined body. The ironic part is she has erected a huge barrier between herself and the key to her thinness: her own body. Communication between an ex-dieter and her body can be re-established, but it takes time, effort, and the new-found trust that comes with understanding.

EMERGENCY SYSTEMS

The human body is equipped with all kinds of emergency systems for adaptation to the limitations of the environment. Unfortunately, we have learned to overuse and abuse these delicate systems by chronically forcing our bodies to cope with unsatisfied physical needs. This is unnecessary in most instances, but because we are so oriented to convenience and technology, we often do not bother with our bodies' "nasty natural functions" at the hint of a need. Stalling until our bodies cannot wait any longer or until it's convenient for us to act, we force our bodies to tolerate much unnecessary stress and we grossly overuse its adaptive mechanisms. We are bound to suffer some bad side effects of this abuse.

BODY ABUSE

Constipation is more common than the common cold! People do not have time to go to the bathroom. They are embarrassed to excuse themselves from a meeting or a social meal. They are rushing around when their colons are trying to work. Frantic physical activity and bowel movements aren't very compatible unless there's diarrhea, which is another way the body copes.

These same people are perplexed and disgusted because they are chronically or intermittently constipated. They get mad at their bodies for this uncomfortable and troublesome quirk. They go to the doctor and get a diagnosis—sluggish colon, spastic bowel, primary congenital constipation. What they really have is a bad case of body abuse from a low-fiber, anti-bread diet (even whole-grain breads are feared by dieters), painfully little physical activity, and loads of mental stress. These people have a lot to learn. They need to listen to their bodies' needs and then respond in normal, appropriate, sympathetic ways.

Suppose someone bought a new car, but she decided that it was too inconvenient to check and change the oil, so she never did it. When her shiny new car breaks down, the engine irreparably burned out, she comes to you, infuriated with the manufacturer at building such an undependable piece of junk. What do you suppose you'd say to her? Touché.

REAL EMERGENCIES

Fatigue, pain, urges, inclinations, appetites, and hunger are all body signals to communicate its needs. Inevitably everybody has to put up with a delay in response to these signals at times. Occasionally, the body has to withstand some unmet needs for longer periods of time. In these special situations, the body uses its built-in emergency systems to adapt to the long- or short-term frustration. This is what they are for—special emergency use when immediate gratification is impossible.

The person who forces her body to habitually overuse and abuse these systems will suffer physical and psychological consequences, but she has no room to complain. When the overweight dieter, for example, consistently tries to ignore her body's fuel-need signal of hunger, her self-defeating habit results in fatigue, headache, irritability, malaise, poor concentration, and exaggerated hunger. She often suffers long-term symptoms, too, including weight gain, digestive trouble, overeating, all sorts of chronic and acute illnesses, as well as a vast array of emotional disturbances. Her body is not the problem. Her misunderstanding is the problem.

MAINTENANCE MATTERS

The woman with the new car and the obese dieter are both missing an important principle—maintenance. Since maintenance is vital to any product's proper functioning and longevity, it is always described in detail in the manufacturer's handbook.

In the case of the car owner, the handbook might have kept her from ruining her car if she had read it, understood its importance, and followed its instructions. But since she refused to respond to the warning light or follow the maintenance instructions, her car broke down, much to her disgust.

The overweight person (and every person) has "warning lights," too. One of them is hunger. If she tries to ignore it, other signals of malfunction will follow: fatigue, headache, etc. The car without oil goes through comparable stages of engine disturbance: rough idle, poor starting, bad odor, and unusual noises. Both "machines" manage to keep going under less-than-ideal conditions, but they will both suffer costly consequences for their owners' negligence.

Ironically, the car and the body are likely to be labeled lemons and rejected by their owners and others alike. Of course, the whole story is never told, and the main results are prejudice and misunderstanding. Interestingly, the manufacturer in each case is often blamed, too, for building such a supposedly inferior product. This is why warrantees do not apply where consumer abuse or neglect have contributed to the product's malfunction.

LIMITED LIABILITY

Manufacturers are obligated to provide a handbook or pamphlet which describes the proper operation and care of their products. Consumers are obliged to read and comply with the instructions, or there is no guarantee, written or understood. If a manufacturer fails to provide such a handbook, he is liable for product malfunction, even if the consumer abuses or fails to maintain the product. But when instructions for use and maintenance are provided yet ignored the product will likely fail or malfunction, especially if it is a sensitive and complicated product like the human body.

GETTING SIGNALS STRAIGHT

Feelings of hunger in general, and most often hunger for pleasure foods can be the body's mistaken signal for other physical needs like rest or sleep, fluids, or physical activity. We are complicated creatures. No wonder we get the signals mixed up sometimes.

DECODING FUEL NEED SIGNALS

My three-year-old son, Michael, provided a beautiful example of this type of mixup one day when he came home from a friend's house at his usual naptime. The first thing he said to me once inside the door was, "Can I have a piece of candy?" We had hard candies left over from Christmas, and he occasionally asks for a piece, so this wasn't unusual.

I knew he was tired because of the time, yet he was telling me about another need. I checked on the possibility of real hunger first, accepting his request as legitimate. "Sounds like you're hungry. You can have a piece of candy after your nap. Would you like a banana?" (A banana is a wonderful, sweet, real food.)

"No!" he protested. "I want a piece of candy!" He meant it, too.

But I wasn't convinced that his need was for candy, so I tried another angle—thirst. "Would you like a glass of orange juice?" I asked. "Yeah," He giggled, "I want a glass of orange juice, and a banana." So he had some juice and a banana and went to bed. He was asleep in five minutes.

Children don't always mean exactly what they say. Who does? When you aren't sure about any person's real message, check it out. Ask some questions. Tell them what you think they mean, but stay open to the possibility of being wrong. Sometimes, every once in a while, your children will ask if they can have cookies, and you can believe that's exactly what they want. Sometimes.

SATISFY THE REAL NEED

If you've got quite a long way to go before a meal (an hour is a long way), and you're tired but not really hungry, drink a glass of cold water and lie down, even on the floor, for just a few minutes. Sleep if possible. You may be tempted to take some pleasure food and coffee, tea, or cola to drink, but that's not a good idea because you're completely missing your body's real need. It isn't smart to have a sweet and a stimulant. You already know it isn't going to solve anything, and it may add to your body's stress. Sugar and caffeine can help you feel better temporarily, but they can really let you down later, especially if you're tired. Water (or any non caffeinated beverage) and rest will have a less dramatic but longer, more comfortable effect.

HUNGRY OR THIRSTY?

Why the water? Thirst, the body's signal for dehydration, sometimes feels a lot like hunger. I think many people eat ice cream and drink pop because of this need mixup. They eat salty food, drink too little fluid with or after the meal, and later, they crave ice cream or pop. Really, they want and need the cold wetness of these pleasure foods, but they would be better satisfied with a glass of ice water. Ice cream and pop are inappropriate.

The body may also crave sweetness because of its need for fat, but once you're off the Feast-or-Famine Cycle, a glass of ice water will sometimes look perfect to you. Then you will be better able to figure out exactly what your body needs. Sometimes, it will be water and a nap.

♣

BREAKFAST

Breakfast is said to be the most important meal of the day. Even if you don't agree now, you may change your mind after you read this section. Early hours and early eating behavior have a powerful effect on your overall eating and weight problem. "But I'm not hungry in the morning!" you protest. Please read on.

The chronic dieter is usually not very hungry when she first gets up in the morning. This is one of the reasons she does her best dieting then. She is not in any real pain without food until later in the day. The other reason that morning dieting is so popular is that hunger is easier to handle when you aren't tired, too.

But if your days of chronic dieting are over and you're determined to break the Feast-or-Famine Cycle, where do you start? In the morning.

Don't Skip Breakfast Anymore. Eat Two!

Don't start by eating a big breakfast. At first, you won't be hungry enough for a big breakfast, anyway, because of your tendency to eat most of your food later in the day. Your body isn't used to getting food in the morning, so it has probably stopped sending signals then. So start by eating some real food that you like as soon as you do get a little hungry in the morning. Eat as much as you need to feel full and satisfied—no more, no less. The tendency is to eat *too little* at this time because of years and years of trying to save calories for later when you are starving. But you aren't going to let yourself get that hungry again, so don't conserve in the morning. You have eaten enough when food doesn't look appealing to you anymore, and if you eat to that point, you may be surprised at how much food you *can* eat. Don't overeat to prevent a hunger pang before lunch. Remember, if you get hungry again before lunch, which is likely, you will eat then, too.

DON'T MAKE RULES

The whole point is, try to stop thinking about amounts and shoulds and shouldn'ts. You may be surprised at how little food it takes to really satisfy you when you're eating the foods you really want to eat. Don't worry about it. Your body knows what it's doing. Your job is to get out of the way. Otherwise you will always need to be fat.

Your need for fat and the consequent overeating of fat-producing foods will not vanish instantly when you begin to apply these principles. Your current need for fat has been established by your past eating behavior of feasts and famines. If you have just been on a very restrictive diet and have lost weight, your body needs to replace those lost fat stores right now. Your tendency, then, will be to overeat and to choose richer, fat-producing foods to make up for the famine your body just went through. You will gain weight at first, perhaps as much as you just lost, but your body will gradually lose its need for excess fat as you eat well. Weight loss *will* follow.

THE NEED TO OVEREAT DISAPPEARS GRADUALLY

When you have eaten enough to feel content, stop eating. This will be easy because food will not appeal to you anymore. If it still looks good, you have probably not eaten enough. You are still coming out of the Feast-or-Famine Cycle, and your body is signalling, by your appetite or food desire, that you need to continue to eat beyond your "hunger." This overeating is caused by past undereating. It will gradually go away as you break the Cycle, but first you must listen carefully to your body's signals, even the overeating ones, and eat more until you want to stop. Don't worry. At some point you will want to stop, and then it will be easy. Little willpower is necessary. You are simply doing what you and your body want to do. Isn't it different?

The next time you feel hungry, eat again. Eat real food that you like until you are satisfied. When you are full, you will know. Stop eating. You know that when you get hungry again, you will eat again, so you don't have to eat in advance of your hunger. Having completely satisfied your hunger from the early part of the day, you won't have to catch up. You are finally beginning to eat according to your body's immediate needs only, thus eliminating its need to store fat for the future.

FOLLOW DIRECTIONS

Each time your hunger signals begin, follow the directions in the last paragraph. They are simple, natural instructions for becoming thin and staying that way. They do not require extraordinary willpower. They do not require special dietary foods. They do not confine your hunger to mealtimes or food-exchange lists.

These instructions are so comfortable and natural that people cannot believe they can lead to anything so wonderful as thinness, but they do. I have seen it happen to ordinary fat people like you and me. And that's why I'm not an ordinary fat person anymore. I'm naturally thin! You can be, too.

OVEREATING AND BINGING STOP

Gradually, as you eat according to your body's fuel-need signals, your nighttime binging and overeating will stop. You will not need to overeat then because you will have supplied your body's fuel needs all day long. You will not feel excessively hungry at night. You will not get overwhelmed by the "munchies". You will not find yourself eating from boredom or tension because your body will not require you to eat when you have no real physical need. It will not need an excuse to get its needs met.

Eating from these other pressures is simply your own interpretation of your body's physical need for make-up food. Munching away compulsively at popcorn or chips in front of the TV is often nothing less than your body's survival instincts in action. Stop blaming your emotions for all your overeating and binging. Most often it's your starving body that gets the munchies. Your emotions shouldn't take the blame.

As your night eating tapers off because of your new eating-by-hunger habits, you will go to bed with an emptier stomach. You will not go to bed hungry because if you are hungry at bedtime, you will eat something. But usually, if you have eaten enough throughout the day (real, quality food), you will not want to eat as often or as much before bed. Chronic dieters have a terrible time imagining this happening to them because they have felt so hungry at night for so long. It does happen, though, even to the die-hard Feast or Faminers. This shift in eating patterns is an important signal that the Cycle is being broken.

Going to bed satisfied but relatively empty, your body has a chance to rest more completely. It does not have half the refrigerator to digest! You will not have gas pains to wake you. You will not sleep so fretfully, working on the pint of ice cream that followed the salty potato chips after your dry, broiled-fish dinner, no potato. Your digestive tract will have a chance to relax too, and while it is relaxing, where is your body's fuel coming from? Your fat will quietly be used for fuel while you sleep, naturally, and painlessly.

BREAKFAST OF THIN CHAMPIONS

Since you have been on a natural mini-fast all night, you will be hungry in the morning. You will want and need to break the fast, so you will eat. You may eat what you used to consider a big breakfast, or it might be quite moderate.

Some people feel a little nauseated after a whole night of fat burning, so they need something light like orange juice, toast, and perhaps fruit. Other popular light breakfasts include things like cereals, toast, muffins, juices, and tea. Sometimes these are the foods that will most appeal to you.

Other favorite breakfast foods are hearty: eggs, ham, cheese omelets, sausage, and rich coffee with cream. Sometimes, after a night of comfortable fasting, you will want these foods for breakfast.

And there will be times when you will want or need two breakfasts in the early hours of the day—one light, just to get you started, and a heavier one later in the morning. Once you are off the Feast-or-Famine Cycle, you can safely eat any real foods your body wants at any time you are hungry. You will learn to trust your body completely, and you will grow slim.

Breakfast will become a very important meal for you because of the benefits of satisfying your morning hunger. You may begin to understand why some nutrition-conscious people say that breakfast is the most important meal of the day. It could be true if it helps you become the thin person you've always wanted to be.

SCHEDULES: NO TIME TO EAT

Many people do not eat well at breakfast. Even nondieters experience lesser weight problems because of careless morning eating. These people don't get hooked on the Cycle of serious undereating and overeating, but they suffer with perhaps ten or fifteen pounds they just can't lose.

Dieters, because of their common heavy night eating and consequent low morning hunger, do their best undereating early in the day.

Besides, who has time to eat a big breakfast? Or any breakfast? Actually, most people don't give themselves time because they don't realize how important it is to eat well in the morning. Besides, they aren't *that* hungry.

If these people began to eat according to their bodies' hunger signals, their morning appetites would gradually become significant enough to compel them to make time for eating before starting the day. They would get up more alert (a benefit of night fasting), and they would make sure to have breakfast because they would be *quite* hungry. Sometimes they would be downright ravenous. These are powerful sensations, even in the sleepiest person.

SPARE TANKS

You wouldn't take your car out for a long drive, knowing that your fuel gauge registered near empty. You could run out of fuel and be stranded. So, since you didn't fill up the night before, you go to the gas station first to ensure that you won't run out of gas.

Yet many people go out in the morning, expecting to use their bodies for transportation, with their fuel gauges near empty. And they do run out of fuel. Because their bodies are equipped with spare fuel tanks (fat) and emergency systems for keeping the ready fuel available for the bodies' needs, they do not get stranded. But their bodies do learn that it's important to keep those spare tanks filled up since the regular tank (stomach) runs on low so much. Once fuel-empty, their bodies begin to use the spare fuel in their muscles and fat.

When these bodies do get a chance to fill-er-up, they

make sure to fill the regular tank and the spare tanks too. They depend on these extra fuel resources for their survival when external fuel is apparently not available. The sad thing is, the fuel (food) is there, but people won't take the time or bother with their bodies' needs. They take better care of their cars.

FILL 'ER UP!

If you are abusing your emergency fuel systems by forcing your body to run on empty, maintain spare fuel tanks, and burn fuel that is supposed to be reserved only for real emergencies, learn to fuel up in the morning. At first a little ready fuel when you get near empty will do, but eventually, you will be able to fill your body's regular tank every day before you take it out for a drive. When that happens, your body can use the spare tank up. After all, you won't be needing it anymore. Besides, it's just been taking up valuable back-seat space.

OVERWEIGHTS WHO DON'T DIET

People who are overweight sometimes swear that they never diet, so how does the Feast-or-Famine Theory apply to them? They are overweight, they say, because they eat too much, and the wrong kinds of food. They have never dieted in their lives, so where's the famine? Is theirs a perennial feast?

Although these people don't actually go on and off traditional diets, the eating-avoidance that traditional diet literature promotes has its subtle effect on their eating behavior. Down deep they believe they are fat because they eat too much, so it makes sense that they should at least try not to eat—and when they do eat, try not to eat so much. They, too, are secretly afraid of eating. They may not be dieting, but they seldom eat when they are just hungry (I call this eating on time). They eat too late. Plain old hunger doesn't justify eating when you are fat, they think. You have to be starving to be able to eat. And starving is excessive hunger, and that's a famine.

Eating late, like dieting, causes obesity. So try eating on time for a change.

EATING OUT

If you have learned to trust your body and to eat according to its needs and appetites, the important thing about eating a meal out will be the fact that you're out. The eating will simply be a nice accompaniment to getting away from the usual home routine.

The body of the chronic Feast-or-Famine dieter, with a little rationalization from the dieter herself, often uses a special occasion where food is a part of the celebrating, to start the feasting part of the Cycle. Sometimes, the dieter consciously plans to overeat, if only just a little. But whether there is premeditation or not, if the current diet has been strenuous and at all "successful", the overeating is seldom just a little. It is typically a true binge, out of the dieter's control—unsatisfying, perplexing, discouraging and certainly fat producing. Having successfully broken down the maladaptive will of the obese undereater, the body now begins the task of replacing the lost fat and possibly adding new for the famines of the future.

The self-effacing, defeated dieter believes that she simply used the picnic, party, or anniversary dinner to

satisfy her sick lust for food. She is deceived. It is her
body's need for fat that has become the overriding influence in restarting the feasting time, and there is honestly nothing she can do about it.

PERMISSION TO EAT PLENTY EVERY DAY

When you eliminate the chronic undersatisfied hunger problems of intermittent dieting, you don't need an
excuse to eat well. You will be eating well all the time,
and slowly losing weight too until you level off slim.

When you go out to eat, you will have the freedom
that all thin people enjoy when they go out for a meal.
You will be able to get anything you are hungry for: lasa-
gna, chicken crepes, steak and baked potatoes. You will
be able to decide more easily what you are hungry for
because you won't be too hungry to think.

You will be able to skip an appetizer because you are
not hungry enough to want or need one, not because
you can't afford the calories. You will be able to have
some hors d'oeuvres when you need a lift before the
main course arrives. You can have a salad with bleu
cheese dressing. You can skip the salad. You can eat
everything on your plate and order more, or you can eat
a little entree and a lot of the exceptional bread. You
can have dessert because you have a craving, or you can
turn it down because you are perfectly satisfied already.
You can own your diet when you eat out, too.

When you plan to eat out, don't save up any of your
hunger for the special meal. Extra hunger isn't what you
need to give you the freedom to eat well. You already
have that freedom and you will enjoy a special eating
occasion much more without feeling overly hungry.

SPOIL YOUR APPETITE

If I'm quite hungry I always eat something substantial
before I go out to eat: half a sandwich, soup, cereal. I

know it will be a while before the food is actually served, and I want to be able to think clearly when I order. I don't worry about spoiling my appetite. That's my goal. Spoiling my appetite is what keeps me thin. And it will make and keep you thin, too.

Regarding wasting food, I know this bothers many people, especially when they eat out. Food waste is often a problem for overweight dieters, especially. Perhaps it is more difficult to throw food away when you are so often going hungry. Thin people who own their own diets don't commonly suffer from food-waste pangs like hungry fat people. So start eating well, and your disposal switch will probably get easier and easier to use.

As for wasting food out, a meal costs the same whether you eat it or not. Try to order according to your appetite. If you're not very hungry and you have a friend along, remember that one shared meal costs half as much as two. But don't forget to tip for two. And doggie bags are for people, too.

THE FOOD AVAILABILITY FACTOR (FAF)

Food availability simply refers to the foods that are available to eat from moment to moment. Food availability answers the question, "What have we got to eat around here?" Why does this FAF need to be controlled? Isn't your body supposed to be in control?

Your body always has an adaptive potential to eat in excess, quantitatively and/or qualitatively, depending on environmental influences. The food availability of the environment is one of those influences. The other is the famine experience. Just as undereating (famine) can stimulate overeating, interest in fat-producing foods, and weight gain, certain foods themselves also stimulate the adaptive potential to overeat and store fat. These foods, usually pleasure foods, are highly refined, having a high proportion of simple carbohydrates (sugars) and fat. They are typically poor in quality for meeting the body's needs.

When pleasure foods are readily available in the environment, you are likely to eat them inappropriately for your body's needs. This is a simple but important truth. And when pleasure foods are not available in your environment (because you did not buy them at the grocery store or pack them in your lunch), you are likely to eat the real foods that are available (because you did buy and pack them). You will eat what you have. Take great care in what you keep (and don't keep) on hand!

Remember, quantity of real food eaten should not be externally controlled. Eliminating excess hunger will naturally lead to appetite adjustment and weight loss. The FAF involves the quality of the diet—the kinds of foods you give your body to meet its fuel needs. Getting off the Feast-or-Famine Cycle will decrease the appetite for pleasure foods, but you must still carefully restrict their availability, at least for the first few months.

THE BUTS

Some overweight dieters protest when I discuss the strict control of pleasure foods. These people, especially homemakers, feel that it's sacrilegious to completely eliminate sweets, treats, and goodies from their homes. They love to bake, they say, for the family, of course. (Do they love being fat?) How can they even think of depriving their children and husbands of these special snacks made with mother's tender loving care?

I'll tell you. They make a choice. They face the reality of their former vulnerability to these goodies. They become honest for a change and courageously do some-

thing for themselves, something much more valuable
than providing pleasure food to those who don't need it
any more than they. After the initial shock, everybody
wins.

Can the high availability of pleasure foods alone promote obesity? Are there people who are fat just because
they eat too much of these foods? Yes and no. People
whose diets are high in poor-quality pleasure foods experience qualitative famines. Food is always there to satisfy hunger signals, but it doesn't meet the body's needs
very well. Their bodies get calories (units of usable energy) all right but very poor nutrition.

Diets high in pleasure foods also inhibit the body's
ability to sense and communicate its needs. In a way,
pleasure foods overload the body's communications
network. It's like putting diesel fuel into a gas-powered
engine. There's bound to be trouble. Big trouble.

EATING FOR OTHERS

Unless you are pregnant or have a tiny baby, you are
not responsible for anyone's body but your own. And,
except for physical safety, you are not even responsible
for your children's bodies, once they are capable of feeding themselves. You are certainly not responsible for
your husband's body, your wife's body, or your neighbor's body either. If you are trying to be responsible for
other people's bodies, read this carefully.

It is infuriating to have well-meaning people encourage me to eat beyond my appetite limits. It is a breach of
trust and love. Should they feel good when I feel terrible
after stuffing myself? When I say that I'm full, they
apparently think I am lying. "But you haven't eaten *that*
much," they insist. I have eaten exactly enough for me,
and that's why I have stopped. I do not believe in saving
room for dessert when I really prefer and need more
real food.

After they question my honesty and perhaps my motives ("Oh, *you* don't need to diet!"), they put the pressure on. It's incredible. "I cooked this dessert especially for you, she'll say. I know how much you like strawberries, so I searched and searched for the recipe. I knew I had it somewhere. I was so relieved to find it. It was a little more complicated to make than I had remembered, but I think it'll be all right. Are you sure you won't have some, for me?"

Holy toledo, if I don't, I'll have to do penance for a month! I want to scream, "No, I won't have some for you! Have some for yourself. I don't eat for other people!"

CHAPTER 7
SPECIAL EFFECTS:
GENDER, METABOLISM,
EXERCISE AND
WOMEN'S SPECIAL TIMES

GENDER DIFFERENCES IN DIETING

Men have a reputation for being able to lose weight much easier than women. Is this true? Women complain that all their husbands have to do is cut down on their eating! They don't have to *starve* themselves like their female counterparts. Why is this? Is there any justice? Is there a sound explanation?

First, is this true? In my observation, it is true that men generally lose weight more readily than women. There are a number of good reasons for this and I have briefly discussed them in Ch. 4. Now let's look more carefully at these influences on the sexes.

Please keep in mind that these explanations are broad generalizations and do not apply to everyone. There are always exceptions.

WHY MEN LOSE WEIGHT MORE READILY THAN WOMEN:

1. Men are not as enslaved by the cultural standards of thinness as women are. They do not panic over a few extra pounds and start a crash diet like many women do. Diets, especially extreme ones, are the starting point of the Feast-or-Famine Cycle. The Cycle creates a need for fat and a resistance to giving it up.

2. Men have naturally higher metabolisms. Perhaps because of this, they do not tolerate prolonged periods without eating as many dieting women do. While women often skip meals altogether, dieting men may eat lighter, but they eat something. Men's famines are not as severe, so their need for fat is not as great, and they are able to give it up more easily.

3. Women have a higher natural affinity for fat because their bodies' survival depends on fat to nourish offspring. Their bodies hold on to fat and resist giving it up because of the biological role of motherhood.

4. Men's metabolic rates probably do not drop as dramatically as women's when they diet. Women's bodies really conserve when their eating is restricted.

5. Men are not as obsessive about weighing themselves. It seems that they lose more quickly because they do not monitor their weight as often.

6. Women, especially right before their periods, tend to retain fluid. Even when they are actually losing fat, the scale does not reflect the loss until the fluid retention shifts. This sets them up for discouragement and severe food restriction.

7. Women have menstrual cycles. Men don't. This

cycle has a notorious effect on diets, eating behavior, and emotions.

MEN AND THE FEAST OR FAMINE CYCLE

Still, men do diet and get caught on the Feast-or-Famine Cycle and gain unattractive weight for many of the same reasons as women.

What hooks men on the Feast-or-Famine Cycle if they don't have the same physiological sensitivities as women? Where do their vulnerabilities lie?

CYCLE STARTERS FOR MEN AND WOMEN ON WORK SCHEDULES

From what men themselves say, limited food availability due to their work schedules seems to be the number one problem. Men generally work away from home where food is not always available. Many women do, too. Working people get hungry at all times of the day, including times when eating is inappropriate if not impossible. Working men and women often skip breakfast or eat very lightly in the morning and they often suffer from excessive hunger by lunchtime. They already have make-up eating to do, and the day is only half done.

Men, like women, are also influenced by traditional diet fallacies and, once a minor weight problem has developed, they begin to consciously watch their weight (control their eating) by avoiding eating and limiting their intake. And so the Cycle starts: undereating followed by overeating. That's all it takes.

What can these people do about their work schedules? One can't just bring out the roast beef on rye in the middle of a math class or a board meeting. And munching a crunchy apple doesn't go well with operating heavy construction machinery or punching computer buttons. How can working people eat whenever they get hungry at work? It takes some planning.

Men, I have found, are often not as interested in planning their eating as women are. This may also make them vulnerable to the Cycle. Wives, mothers, or girlfriends can be helpful in making real food more available to the working man. But avoid being overbearing.

You Can (and Must) Take It With You

First, breakfast is an *absolute must* for people on a work schedule away from home if they want to be thin. Reread the section on breakfast if you wonder why. Portable food can be packed for daytime hunger, and there are usually enough breaks to prevent excessive hunger if breakfast was well eaten. Lunch need not be eaten exclusively at lunchtime. A tuna-salad sandwich might be perfect for the ten o'clock coffee break. Maybe milk and fruit is all that's needed at noon. Or something fresh in the cafeteria may appeal to you at lunchtime. A second sandwich may fill the need/hunger at three and you get home before you feel starved. Always pack more than you (or he) will need. Quality early daytime eating has a dramatic effect on nighttime hunger and eating. That's how the Cycle can be broken and where thinness can begin.

BURNING IT OFF WITH EXERCISE: EXPOSING THE MYTH

My son has a tee shirt with a photo of a jogger on it. It says, "Burn It Off". This phrase reflects a common misconception about exercise and fat. In reality, fat does not burn off during exercise. There are many other physiological effects of exercise, but fat burning is not one of them. The things that exercise does burn are calories, most of them from ready blood glucose and glycogen stores, not fat. But the "bad news" is that relatively few calories are burned over time, even during vigorous exercise. This reflects the efficiency of the human body and is really a good thing.

Some of the important benefits of regular exercise include:

1.   Shapes up your cardiovascular system.
2.   Stimulates your metabolism.
3.   Makes you feel better, increases health and energy.
4.   Improves your overall appearance.
5.   Increases your stamina.
6.   Improves muscle tone.
7.   Promotes sound and efficient sleep.

The list could be longer but weight loss would not be an appropriate addition. Exercise does not cause weight loss primarily. Exercise stimulates the metabolic rate, which, coupled with a high quality diet can lead to a trimmer figure. But this is a secondary effect. Perhaps people who exercise regularly feel freer to eat more, and that is definitely a plus.

WHY OVERWEIGHT PEOPLE AVOID EXERCISE

Knowing all the beneficial effects of regular exercise, why don't more people do it? Why don't more overweight people, especially, get out and exercise? Are they just lazy?

From what we already know about the body's survival drive and its effect on our eating behavior, is there something about exercise and being overweight that doesn't mix well? Yes. And I believe it explains much of the movement-resistance that overweight people experience.

When a body's survival depends on storing and conserving fat, and it is working very hard to achieve these goals, wouldn't unnecessary activity be counterproductive? Think about it. And since the body inspires behaviors that lead to fat storage and conservation (overeating, interest in fat-producing foods, etc.) doesn't it make sense that the overweight person would be motivated *by need* to avoid excess movement? It makes sense to me.

BMR (BASAL METABOLIC RATE)

This is a medical term which refers to the speed at which your body hums along in neutral. There is a range of low to high, like the normal cool-to-medium-hot range at which engines normally run. If you are concerned about your BMR you can have it checked by your doctor.

EXERCISE AND WHAT?

There are two natural ways to stimulate your metabolic rate. You probably know the first one—exercise. Increasing your activity level does stimulate your metabolism. And that higher metabolic rate stays higher even after you quit exercising. The other natural way to raise your metabolism is not commonly known—eating. Eating?

Yes. Eating stimulates your metabolism. Your body's engine burns hotter and faster when you eat regularly. And the reverse is also true: When you don't eat regularly, your metabolism slows down. Your engine stays cooler in order to conserve energy. This makes sense because your body cannot afford to waste any fuel when there's no fuel available. What if you really got stranded without food? If your body continued to burn hot and fast you would not survive very long. Remember that your body's primary job is to keep you alive.

In college, when I was dieting all the time, my BMR was tested. It was low, but within the normal range despite my relatively high activity level. I walked miles to class every day and often played tennis. I now believe my poor eating habits contributed to my sluggish BMR. In fact, the effect of my eating habits were more powerful than the stimulating effect of the exercise.

Now my BMR is much closer to the middle of the normal range even though I exercise less. My hands and feet are warm now, I eat twice as much on a regular basis, and I am thin.

EXERCISE AND DIET

Without a high-quality diet, an exercise program can make a famine even more stressful to the body. The poor-quality, traditional weight-loss diet plus exercise creates a physiological catastrophe—a severe famine. This famine with increased, often strenuous, activity is extremely stressful to the body. The body is forced to adapt to two major physical stressors—poor food availability and physical exertion. One without the other is bad enough, but together they are disastrous.

Often the body acquiesces and gives up its energy stores. Remember, once the liver's glycogen stores are used up the body breaks down muscle—not fat—when it needs energy in a hurry. The internal organs and body muscle are used for quick energy. The person on such a program loses pounds and may lose them fast since glycogen and muscle are weighty compared to bulkier, lighter fat tissue.

For a time there may be a dramatic weight loss while the body scrambles to survive and stay healthy. Along with this weight-and-water loss come other much less desirable symptoms: fatigue, muscle weakness, headache, nausea, excessive hunger, and restlessness. Who can keep it up? Not too many bodies can or will.

OWN YOUR EXERCISE, TOO

Like your eating program, a successful exercise program should be very personal. You must choose it for yourself, guided if necessary by your physician. In exercise, like your eating, you must listen carefully to signals from your body and heed them. Your body has important information for you if you will just tune in to it. This doesn't mean you shouldn't push your body at times. It does mean that you must begin gradually and build your body up with care. It is a fine and delicate instrument.

THE MOVEMENT MOTIVE

Most people misunderstand exercise. Exercise is simply physical activity. An exercise program may be something quite different, but plain old exercise is something everybody who moves does. In order to increase your exercise, all you have to do is move more. Now this sounds simple but it's not. Moving more is usually a problem unless you *have to* move more. If you were hired tomorrow to load potatoes onto semis, you'd be exercising in a hurry. The movement motive would be built into your job.

Well, you're probably not loading potatoes, so how do you get the movement motive into your lifestyle so exercise can be a more natural part of your life? Look around you. Discover motives to move. Then arrange your environment so that you have to move more to live.

Here are some examples of motivated movement:

1. Rent a parking space in a lot six blocks from your

workplace.
2. Keep the laundry room at least one story away from your living areas.
3. Store firewood in the basement for upper floor fireplaces or vice versa.
4. Use only one phone in your house or apartment whenever possible. Keep it in the farthest corner from where you spend most of your time.
5. Don't keep everything at your desk within reach. Store occasional essentials across the room, or better still, across the hall.

In theater, there must be a motive for every move on stage. It's the same for exercise. So work the motives into your lifestyle, and your lifestyle will work you into better shape.

EXERCISE AND PAIN

There is one other misconception about exercise that deserves a comment because it keeps people from getting into shape. It is the idea that physical activity must be vigorous and sweat producing in order to qualify as genuine exercise. This isn't true. In fact, most real exercise is not particularly strenuous. It feels rather natural and comfortable. We are made with motion in mind, and it makes sense that moving around shouldn't usually hurt. If it does, sooner or later we'll probably give it up. Pain and survival are not close friends.

The point is, if you want to move more for your body's sake, make the moving you do enjoyable. It should feel good most of the time. Now I know some avid runners who admit they hate to run. It hurts, they say. I feel sorry about that because I think there must be a better way for them to move besides running. (The main reason they continue is that they get hooked on the terrific way the running makes them feel afterward.)

It's worthwhile to spend some time investigating different types of activities to find out what you *like* to do. You are most likely to do those things. Make a list and then do the list, little by little. Don't try to do it like the Olympic Triathalon. Just set out to enjoy more often the activities you like, and gradually you'll also be enjoying the good effects of the exercise on your body. It's worth an effort. Remember, you only get one body. You might as well make the most of it.

WOMEN'S EXCLUSIVE TIMES

The rest of this chapter is devoted to some of the particular needs of women. These areas include the physical changes that occur with the monthly period and pregnancy, and the emotional effects of scales and support groups.

WEIGHT FLUCTUATIONS WITH THE MENSTRUAL CYCLE

Women experience slight, natural changes in their day-to-day weight with the menstrual cycle. These shifts upward and downward are caused by two basic factors: hormones which influence salt and fluid retention, and changes in appetite. Actually, appetite changes are also influenced by hormone shifts, so I suppose female hormones can be blamed there, too. I use the word blame because these hormones and their consequent weight fluctuations often discourage the overweight woman and help lead to diet failure. The naturally thin woman hardly notices such variations in appetite and body weight although the familiar bloated feeling sometimes causes complaint.

The increase in appetite that most women experience before their periods is their bodies' way of preparing for possible conception. The same hormones that stimulate appetite in the pregnant woman, estrogen and progesterone, come into play here. Progesterone has the more influential role in premenstrual time and pregnancy. The body is getting ready to nourish a baby, which, to the body of a still-menstruating woman, is always a possibility, regardless of her marital status, sexual involvement, or efforts at contraception. These hormones also promote slight, temporary fluid retention. This also apparently prepares the body for conception, and in that sense is adaptive.

Sometimes, around the onset of menses (a woman's period) the hormones and their effects shift. This shift and the consequent changes in appetite and body hydration are comparable to the changes of a normal woman postpartum (after birth). Of course, they are not nearly as dramatic, but they do compare in the natural elimination of excess fluid by the kidneys. Also, the appetite drops off rather suddenly, leaving a natural, comfortable, empty feeling. The body feels and is lighter. Sometimes premenstrual fluid retention accounts for a transient weight gain of four or five pounds, but this amount is entirely eliminated once the kidneys get the message from the hormone shift and the period starts beginning another cycle.

CYCLE ON CYCLE

Why is this such a distressful time for the overweight, chronic dieter? Instead of allowing for her body's normal changes in hydration and appetite and accepting the weight gain and extra hunger as normal, the chronic dieter, bent on fast weight loss alone, panics at these changes each month. Because she does not trust her body, she fights her increased appetite, getting hungrier and hungrier, instead of simply eating a little more real food to satisfy her body's increased need. As she resists her body's signals for an increased need for fuel and sticks inflexibly to her diet regimen, she exaggerates the severity of her famine. Often these stresses become overwhelming, and her body breaks into the feasting part of the Cycle at this time of the month.

The picture is grim. The overweight woman on a weight-reduction diet does fairly well for two and a half weeks. She loses perhaps six pounds or more by sheer willpower and self-denial. She grows in courage and self-esteem, day by day, pound by pound. Then all of a sudden, it seems, her appetite goes completely out of control. One morning she finds herself eating sweet rolls, one after another, for no apparent reason. She feels ravenous and very upset. Why can't she stop? When she does stop, after four and a half sweet rolls, (a thousand calories!) she is mortified and frightened.

What happened? Has she lost her grip, her willpower? She is somehow out of that lucky groove she had hoped would last a lifetime this time. She has gone off her diet, and she is ashamed. In the grips of self-pity, guilt, and tremendous post-famine hunger (which always go together), she begins the feasting, rationalizing all the way to the refrigerator. Her body has won the battle.

PREMENSTRUAL BINGING IS UNIVERSAL IN DIETERS

This woman's appetite got the best of her during the week before her period. Many women lose weight quickly and diet fairly successfully during the first three weeks of their menstrual cycles. It's a three-week famine that their bodies have had to adjust to by keeping them overweight. Then, sometime around that fourth week, their bodies' increased fuel needs trigger unbearable hunger.

This is not the normal premenstrual hunger of the naturally thin woman. This excessive, maladaptive hunger is caused by a combination of famine and increased physiological need. It defies the willpower and normal satiation point of the dieter.

Women who are on this three-week/one-week Feast-or-Famine Cycle literally eat more than enough food in one week to make up for three weeks of strenuous dieting. The body has an uncanny ability to adjust to the insanity we impose on it. The saddest part is, these women, for all their efforts, are fat throughout their cycle, getting fatter in the long run, month by month, and suffering all the way.

DON'T PANIC. EAT!

When you learn to trust your body's fuel-need signals, and your appetite increases premenstrually, you will naturally eat more real food. You will be hungry more often, and it will take a little more food to satisfy your hunger completely, which you must do in order to get and stay thin. Besides ensuring your slim figure, a healthy diet during this time will help you feel more relaxed when hormones and body changes often promote tension.

When your period does start, you'll naturally get back to normal within a few days or a week. And don't forget, if a new baby is in the picture, your body has a healthy, slender head start toward a healthy, slender pregnancy!

PREGNANCY

Earlier in the book (Ch. 2) I talked about the menarche, which is the onset of menstruation in girls. This is a very common time for weight-consciousness to begin, and understandably so. About the time of their first periods, girls start to gain weight and develop curves that weren't there before. Their appetites increase, they eat more food, and their bodies deposit fat in certain strategic locations: breasts, hips, tummy, buttocks, and thighs.

There is also more fat deposited all over the body, smoothing out the angular look of younger girls and contrasting the typically lanky look of adolescent boys. These changes are normally slight, quite imperceptible from day to day. All of a sudden, it seems, a girl turns into a woman. But why all these changes?

FAT IN NONPREGNANT WOMEN

A moderate amount of body fat is adaptive (supporting survival) for women of child-bearing age because of the possibility of conception. The early pregnancy nausea many women experience may be due to the stress and change the body is going through to grow a baby. If conception does occur and some appetite suppression follows, these small fat stores are used for fuel at this time of decreased food intake. Healthy, lean women sometimes even lose a little weight during the first few months of pregnancy because of this, and the normal, increased appetite returns about the second trimester (end of the third month). Apparently, the body has made its adjustments by then and is ready to handle more fuel from the environment.

FAT IN EARLY PREGNANCY

The nonpregnant woman keeps a little extra fat all the time, just in case of conception. The newly pregnant woman, if she listens to her body signals, allows that fat to be used while she eats less or lighter foods because of her lesser hunger and/or nausea. (It is also perfectly normal to feel nauseated and still gain weight in the first months of pregnancy. And many women are not nauseated at all.)

But what about later when this pregnant woman becomes ravenous? She apparently needs to eat more, right? That's what the ravenous signal is for. The body is asking for more food. If she responds with sanity, understanding, and faith in her body's signals, she will naturally begin to eat more real food and gradually gain weight. She will feel good. If the ravenous signal causes her to panic, on the other hand, and she tries to diet by trying not to eat, you know she is in trouble.

DIETING DURING PREGNANCY

The stress the dieting pregnant woman puts on her body is enormous. She is pregnant, carrying a developing baby. Her body changes dramatically from month to month. Her metabolic and nutritional needs increase considerably. She is excited and nervous about having a baby. She worries about her husband's fear of the new responsibilities. On top of all this, she starts fighting her body. It's insane.

Fortunately her body's need will override her willpower, and she will probably eat more and gain weight whether she (or her doctor) approves or not. She doesn't need an extra challenge at this time.

THE ROLE OF FAT THROUGHOUT PREGNANCY

An increase in overall body fat for the pregnant woman is adaptive because, in light of the body's life-supporting needs, there's always a chance that the pregnant woman will experience a famine. Or, there's the possibility that the baby will be born during a season of low food availability. In these situations, the mother's body is not only responsible for its own fuel requirements, but it must also provide the fetus or newborn infant's fuel needs.

This natural increase in total body fat should be moderate if the woman is regularly satisfying her body's hunger with real, high-quality food. Adapting to the environment of continuous, quality food supply, her body has no need to store a large amount of food as fat. In other words, the gathering of excess fat against the possibility of famine will be minimal since no famine, real or artificial, occurs during pregnancy.

WHEN OVERWEIGHT DIETERS GET PREGNANT

The strict Feast-or-Famine dieter who gets pregnant presents a totally different picture. Pregnancy often causes a prolonged feast for the serious eating-avoidance dieter. If conception occurs at a time when the dieter has successfully lost a considerable amount of weight, such as twenty or more pounds, or has maintained weight loss by going hungry much of the time, the increased metabolic demands and the post-famine need for fat can send even the most conscientious calorie counter on a nine-month binge. She may try to control her weight by undereating, but that only makes matters worse.

Doctors and midwives are often perplexed when such excessive weight is gained in pregnancy and they counsel their patients to watch their eating. Obesity and pregnancy don't mix very well. But actually, these pregnant women should have been watching their eating long before the pregnancy began. These unhappy women are not weak willed or unmotivated. They are overwhelmed.

ADAPTATIONS DURING NORMAL PREGNANCY AND INFANCY

The pregnant woman normally needs only a little more food, perhaps more often, because her body's needs are greater than before. Her appetite should increase in perfect proportion to her body's needs, and if she listens to her body, she will gain exactly the right amount of weight to ensure a well-nourished, healthy infant and her own postpartum health. She will not have to go on a diet after the baby is born. Her body will gradually use up the extra fat it stored because the need will have passed. And when the need for fat passes, fat naturally disappears, too.

These same principles apply to the fully developed newborn, who also has some fat saved up. There is an interesting delay in milk flow in the new mother after her baby is born. Instead of the breasts producing milk immediately after delivery, their milk production is delayed for a few days. I believe this is also adaptive.

During those first days, the newborn does not get a significant amount of nourishment from the breast. The baby does suck instinctively when put to the breast, but the breast delivers little drops of colostrum instead of milk. Colostrum is important for the baby's resistance to disease. But no milk. Why?

Like its mother's body in early pregnancy, the infant's body is under considerable stress, adjusting to the changes of life outside the womb. Apparently, it doesn't need digestive stress too, so it uses its own internal food supply for a few days, content on colostrum and mother's warm body. The baby loses some weight during this time, but it is prepared to do this by its fat and water reserves. The newborn also dehydrates somewhat, which explains why pregnant women retain fluid (overhydration) and often crave salty foods (promoting fluid retention).

The pregnant woman gets somewhat overhydrated, and the baby is born that way—also overhydrated—to ensure adequate fluid balance until the milk comes in. (Excessive fluid retention is maladaptive and potentially dangerous.) Since dehydration during pregnancy is also potentially hazardous for the fetus and mother, some extra fluid insures against any threatening fluid loss throughout pregnancy. To the body, these things are simply a matter of survival in a changing environment.

The woman who is nursing also experiences a greater appetite than when she wasn't pregnant. Her appetites for certain foods might also be affected by her unique needs during lactation.

CHAPTER 8
PASSING IT ALONG:
CHILDREN AND FAMILIES

FAT ROLES AT DIFFERENT STAGES OF LIFE

Understanding the various roles that fat plays at different stages of life enables you to help yourself and perhaps others to get and stay slim. So whether you have been overweight ever since you can remember or have more recently developed a weight problem, this section will help you find the missing pieces to the obesity puzzle. And if you have children or expect to in the future, this material is vital.

BABY FAT

This term refers to the fat an infant acquires after the newborn stage. Babies have a reputation for being naturally fat, hence the expression, baby fat. If babies are fat by nature, isn't it possible for adults to be naturally fat, too? No, not unless there is disease or real famine.

First of all, babies aren't *that* fat by nature, and the fat they do acquire is almost always adaptive. Babies who are extremely fat are usually very muscular babies. If they are not particularly muscular but just soft and very fat, they could be misfed. They might be put on solid foods with too much pleasure food too soon. They may drink rich formula which does not gradually thin out as the baby finishes drinking like breast milk does. They might be fed inappropriately on too rigid a schedule so that they get too hungry and have to overeat to make it through four hours. Or they might be fed too often, at times when they have other needs like sucking or sleep. And sometimes, mothers' expectations for their babies' eating habits are too rigid. Babies' fuel needs change constantly from day to day, but mothers often think that six ounces, for example, is minimum for a "good meal."

Normal baby fat is different. It is adaptive. A baby's survival depends on fat for several reasons. Babies are helpless, totally dependent on others for food, body warmth, stimulation, and protection. Their baby-fatness between birth and age two or three is adaptive because of this complete dependency.

They need insulation from temperature changes when they kick off their blankets. They need a substantial internal source of food if they get hungry during the night and no one hears them cry or they don't wake up. This same internal source of food must supply their bodies' needs during illness when they cannot or will not eat for several days. Babies also need padding for those inevitable falls. Unquestionably, babies need to be fat. So they generally are.

WHEN AND WHY BABY FAT DISAPPEARS

Interestingly, when babies get to be about two years old (unless they are not allowed to own their diets), they gradually lose their baby fat. Sometimes this happens sooner, sometimes a little later, but it is usually completely gone by the time they are four or five. At the age of two or three, little children are no longer totally dependent. They are able to feed themselves and hopefully have some choice about what they eat and when.

They can obtain food for themselves in a limited but significant way. They can talk or use other signals. They can demand. They can persuade. They are not as vulnerable to baby-type accidents or illness. As their dependency needs for baby fat disappear, the baby fat disappears, too.

Babies trust their bodies. They don't know any better. When they feel hunger, a painful sensation, they cry. They don't think about it, and that's good. If they did, they would fall prey to all the entanglements that we get ourselves into.

If a baby's caretaker, let's say it's Daddy this time, doesn't know what the child's crying means (and it always means something) he might use the trial-and-error method: Change the diaper. That's not it. Try a burp. No, still crying. Gas? Bounce the baby on her tummy. Not that either, and now the baby is not just crying, she is screaming mad.

The baby is not thinking, "Poor Daddy, he's doing the best he can. I should show him that I appreciate his efforts and settle down even though I'm still starving. After all, you can't expect a father to know what to do right off the bat!" Of course the baby is not thinking these things. And that's good because if she quit crying to protect Daddy's feelings, she might starve before Daddy thought of putting a bottle in her mouth.

After all, Daddy is thinking, "It *can't* be hunger. She's not due for another bottle for two hours."

Instead of being placated by Daddy's misguided efforts, the baby cries until she gets exactly what she needs—food. Babies know very little. Their bodies know a lot. They have to trust their bodies. Their survival depends on it, and maybe that's why they don't have a choice.

Unfortunately, we do.

FAT CHILDREN

If you were a fat child, this idea of becoming naturally slim must, in a way, sound like a pipe dream. You must see what happened to your body along the way that caused the fat and kept it going. And if you have children, you can help carve out a new path for them. It is the same road that will lead to your recovery from this life-long curse.

After four or five years of age children are naturally quite lean. They have used up their baby fat, which has become unnecessary as a survival aid. This is true only as long as there is a continuous and adequate supply of food available. Mothers often worry about how to eliminate their children's round cheeks and chubby tummies. They wouldn't have to worry if they understood what is going on in their toddlers and why, and how healthy it really is.

HOW BABY FAT DISAPPEARS

Since baby fat becomes unnecessary with growing independence and physical coordination, the most adaptive response to these changing needs is for the body to eliminate most of it. Instead of having survival benefits, extra fat becomes a burden for the child's body, making it less efficient.

How does the body get rid of it? This is the part that troubles mothers—the child's appetite changes. He gradually becomes finicky about what he eats and when. He develops strong likes and dislikes and literally cannot be forced to eat food he doesn't want. Neither will he eat when he is not hungry. His appetite seems unpredictable and sporatic—sometimes ravenous, sometimes nonexistent. This is universal and normal. The child is owning his diet, something we must all learn to do again.

This last paragraph also describes the appetite

changes that occur in a person getting off the Feast-or-Famine Cycle. The continuous availability of quality food eliminates the need for excess fat. The body adjusts its hunger and fuel-need signals, allowing the elimination of the now burdensome fat. The ex-dieter becomes a picky eater after the Cycle is broken, and her eating is unpredictable and sporatic, complete with cravings (often for specific vegetables or whole-grain bread), and aversions. The changes are rather dramatic. Be ready for them.

WHEN BABY FAT DOESN'T DISAPPEAR

Any child who owns her diet at this stage will lose her baby fat, generally growing taller and slimmer through early grade school. The child who is unable to own her diet, for one reason or another, will not lose her baby fat, and generally will grow taller and fatter through grade school. This is not normal. It's a tragedy. The fat child's whole personality and happiness is often affected by her fatness. She will be forced, during her most formative years, to try to grow up with the handicaps of obesity. She will be rejected, ridiculed, laughed at, and misunderstood. Her friendships will be limited, her whole life confined by her abnormal body.

Sound melodramatic? Then you weren't a fat child, and you've never really known one. Why do some children become fatter when most are growing slim? The reasons are far too complex to cover thoroughly in this book, but I do have some thoughts on this problem.

FAMINE SENSITIVITY IS INHERITED

The Adaptation Theory that I have proposed does not support the notion that obesity is inherited. I do not believe that it is, either. So let's focus on some important environmental influences.

Keep in mind that children do inherit sensitivities to

food availability in the environment. Their bodies are more or less prone to react to famines (unsatisfied hunger) by fat storage because of the influence of their parents' genetic sensitivities.

ENVIRONMENTAL FACTORS THAT AFFECT CHILDHOOD OBESITY

1. Parents of fat children may not own their own diets. That is, they are not in touch with their bodies' needs and signals. If they do not own their diets (which is most likely the case if they are overweight, too), they will not be inclined to allow or encourage their children to own their diets.
2. Parents of fat children may be caught in the Feast-or-Famine Cycle—underfed and overfed. Children get caught in it too, just living in the same house. They copy attitudes and behaviors.
3. Parents offer pleasure foods inappropriately at times when the child's body is signalling for real food. Children get hungry often because they use a lot of energy and are growing fast. They will eat the foods that are consistently made available to them. If it's cookies and potato chips, that's what they'll eat. If it's fruit and peanut-butter sandwiches, that's what they'll eat. What they see is what they'll eat.
4. Quality real foods that children like to eat are not available enough to meet their bodies' needs and fuel-need signals. They substitute poor-quality pleasure foods to make up for insufficient real foods.
5. Parents use food for reward and punishment which pressures the child's eating choices and gives food exaggerated significance for the child.

Food can become to children more than just fuel for the body.

6. Children's eating choices are judged by inappropriate standards. Parents praise and reward children (often with pleasure food) for cleaning their plates, regardless of their bodies' real need for what was on the plates or their desire to stop eating when they felt full.

PARENTS PROMOTE FEAST-OR-FAMINE CYCLE IN CHILDREN

Children learn attitudes and behaviors from their parents. They tend to act and think very much like their parents. If parents have unhealthy ideas about food plus unnatural eating habits, children are likely to suffer the effects of these attitudes and habits, too. In a passive way, these parents pass obesity on to their children.

But there are more active ways of promoting obesity in offspring. Some parents panic about a child's chubbiness. (Children do go through normal chubby stages which they usually outgrow within a year.) But if a parent panics and puts the child on a restrictive diet, the child and eventually the adult she grows into, will probably always be fat.

DON'T WAIST FOOD

By the way, since portions served are not always portions needed, especially with children's unpredictable appetites, won't there be a lot of food wasted?

Wasting food is not a sin. Food wasted in garbage disposals or waste baskets (it might help if you think of it as a "waist" basket) is food much better spent than food wasted on a human body. Food waste is inevitable, one way or another, so if you have to waste it or waist it, waste it for sure!

Whether or not you have a fat child, if you can identify

with some of these fat-promoting factors, think about your attitudes and habits regarding food and eating. You probably learned them from your parents, and they from their parents, and so on. You also learned them from traditional diet literature. In retrospect you can blame ignorance. We all can. But now and in the future there's nothing to blame. We know a better way.

THE BOY AT THE PICNIC

I once met a not-so-little six-year-old boy at a school picnic. He came straight over to me from the big picnic shelter where all the food was set out on tables. Quite outgoing, he smiled and asked if he could join my daughter and me on our picnic blanket. Since he was obviously overweight (children at six are generally on the thin side), I took note of what he was eating. He had a hot dog, potato chips, and a cup of Kool-aid. That seemed normal. As he put his plate down on the blanket, he proudly confided that he'd managed to get another one of the jumbo-size hot dogs. So, this was his second.

That didn't strike me as particularly unusual either, but I couldn't resist asking a few questions. He'd had Rice Krispies for breakfast. So what? My slim daughter had had cold cereal, too, and happens to love Rice Krispies.

All of a sudden this nice little boy got up and bee lined over to the food shelter, returning with two chocolate-frosted brownies. As he started to eat them, I thought. Where's the famine here? Maybe he's an "emotional overeater" although he seemed so emotionally balanced, so friendly and secure. Maybe he just has a naturally big appetite—big parents.

When he returned to the shelter, apparently for another refill, I was having real doubts. It sure seemed like this boy was fat just because he ate so much. Once again he returned to our spot, this time with two Rice Krispies squares. He offered one to my daughter, and she took it eagerly. (That's a big treat for my kids.) He's getting filled up, I thought. But no, back for more brownies a few minutes later. This was turning into serious overeating behavior!

As we chatted between trips, he pointed out his mother to me. She was quite tall, of medium build, perhaps a muscular person, but not fat, not even borderline obese. His little sister was also normal. He shared himself so openly and was so skilled socially for a six-year-old that the more I thought about it, I just couldn't believe he had big emotional problems.

But then, while he finished his fourth rich brownie, he just about knocked me over when he commented, "I'm on a diet."

WHOSE DIET?

Six-year-olds do not go on diets by themselves. And he certainly wasn't supposed to be on a high-calorie diet. Apparently, this boy had been put on a restrictive diet by his concerned parents and doctor. The Feast-or-Famine Cycle was already well established—periods of undereating (dieting) followed by periods of make-up overeating. I caught this boy in the feasting stage, and his body, not his mother, was in control for a change.

PLEASURE-FOOD ABUSE IS COMMON IN KIDS

Just like adults, children can be taught to want foods that their bodies cannot use well. They can actually learn to prefer these foods for inappropriate use to meet their fuel needs. Pleasure foods are often used inappropriately in place of real foods. Cookies are perhaps the most commonly abused pleasure food where children are concerned.

"THE COOKIE CONFLICT"

When a child comes home from school, he is almost always hungry. His body is signaling a need for fuel, and if he owns his diet, he automatically looks for something to eat. There are freshly baked cookies out on the table. Mom has just finished baking them, and the sweet smell fills the entire house. Mom has had a few—just to test for doneness—but she plans to save the rest for dessert. It's 3:45.

Son: "Hey, Mom, can I have a cookie?"

Mother: "Don't touch those cookies. They're for dessert!"

Son: "But I'm hungry!"

Mother: "We're eating in a little while. You'll spoil your dinner."

Son: "But I'm starving!"

Mother: "I don't care. I'm fixing a nice dinner, and I don't want you to fill up on cookies."

Son: "Awe, Mom."

Mother: "O.K., you may have *one*. But I made them for dessert. Go outside. Do your homework. Stop bugging me."

What is happening here? What has provoked such an angry conflict? Miscommunication and misinformation.

FUEL-NEED SIGNAL IN DISGUISE

The missed communication began with the first sentence—"Can I have a cookie?" What is the child really saying? He wants a cookie, but in a broader sense he is communicating a need, a very strong physical need for fuel. Because Mother is unaware of this broader meaning, she responds literally, ignoring the real need behind the request—the need for quality real food. And because that survival-instinct need is so strong, the boy persists, knowing full well that he will probably make his mother angry. Her rejection of him is not even as bad as his hunger at this point.

The boy tries to clarify by protesting her denial: "I'm hungry!" He means that he needs to eat and he needs to eat now.

But mom has other plans that conflict with that need, however strong. Getting closer to his real meaning, she argues that now is not the right time for him to eat because now is not dinnertime. She doesn't believe in eating between meals, however hungry you feel. After all, she goes hungry most of the day. If it doesn't kill her, a little hunger won't hurt him, either.

The statement she makes about eating in a little while is a lie. It is only 3:45 and, as her son well knows, dinner is never ready before 5:30—almost two hours away. Two hours is *not* a little while for any hungry person, especially a child. It is a very long, uncomfortable amount of time.

WHAT'S THE POINT?

"But I'm starving!" gets closer still to his real need, but Mom is still not hearing his need. She is too busy protecting her cookies. Her response, "I don't care," is true, in a way. But her main problem is that she is completely missing her son's point in asking for a cookie in the first place.

♣

"THE COOKIE CONNECTION"

The same scene can be reenacted with new information, better communication, and a happier ending.

Same scene and characters:

Son: "Hey, Mom, can I have a cookie?"

New Information: When a person asks for something sweet, it often signals a need for real food

Mother: "Sounds like you're hungry."

Better communication: When you think a person is communicating something more than the literal meaning, first find out if your hunch is true.

Son: "Yeah, I'm starved. The heat went out in the school building, so we got to play basketball in the gym all afternoon. It was great!"

New information: There is always a good reason for hunger. Extra physical activity is one of them. Hunger demands satisfaction.

Mother: "You must be starved. Have a cookie while I fix you something more solid to eat. What would you like?"

Better communication and new information: Cookies are OK for fast relief, but they cannot satisfy fuel needs very well. Real food will better satisfy the body's needs. Hunger for pleasure foods or sweets usually means the body needs real food.

Son: "Thanks." He takes a cookie. "A roast-beef sandwich would be great. I could eat two!"

New information: Excess hunger often requires extra food. This is the body's normal way of making up for missed fuel.

Mother: "I'll bet you could. I'll fix one now, and it'll probably hold you off til dinner. We'll eat right on time tonight because I'm sure you'll be hungry again by then."

Son: "Thanks alot, Mom." He takes the sandwich.

"This'll be O.K. for now. What are we having for dinner?"

Mother: "Spaghetti, your favorite."

Son: "Great. Can I have a glass of milk?"

Mother: "Sure."

PEANUT-BUTTER-AND-JELLY SANDWICHES

If you took a poll of children's all-time, all-American, over-all favorite main course or lunch-box item, the overwhelming majority vote would be for the classic peanut-butter-and-jelly sandwich.

It's my three-year-old's favorite. He prefers a peanut-butter-and-jelly sandwich over grilled cheese. He wants it more than bologna with mayo. He'll even take it in lieu of his favorite dinner, spaghetti.

I have never heard a hungry child refuse one. Why?

Judging from what I know of physiology, metabolism, and human fuel requirements, the peanut-butter-and-jelly sandwich is a stroke of nutritional genius. It combines in a delicious, easy-to-handle, adhesive, and portable food, a perfect combination of rich energy fuels. The jelly provides immediate blood-sugar elevation, relieving the child's anxious appetite. The peanut butter is loaded with nutrients: vitamins, minerals, protein for growth, fat for stable energy fuel, roughage, and ready carbohydrates. And bread, especially whole-grain bread, is also a terrifically nutritious food. What more can you ask for? Just a glass of milk.

Children love peanut-butter-and-jelly sandwiches, and that's why. If you still doubt whether you can really trust your child's body to desire the right foods in the right amounts at the right time, read this section again. You

may even consider having a PB and J sandwich yourself.
They're great!

OTHER PEOPLE'S DIETS

Please do not try to inflict your own needs on other
people at the expense of their comfort. It isn't nice and
they won't like you for it.

If you are trying to control what your children eat, you
are wasting a lot of emotional energy because your efforts are aimed in the wrong direction. Your children
will eat the foods that are made available to them when
they are hungry. Please read that sentence again because we're going to break it down and study it.

Your children. They are not you or even extensions of
you. They are separate people, other people. Since a
person cannot eat for other people, at least not literally,
they should not eat for the sake of other people's needs,
figuratively speaking.

Will eat. Healthy children of any age do not have to be
coaxed or forced to eat unless they are not hungry. They
have strong survival instincts and eating food to satisfy
hunger is one of their major drives.

The foods that are made available to them. Are you
ready, Mom, Dad? This is where you come in. You are
the ones who make food available at home. You buy the
groceries. You fix the meals. (More on this later because
it is the only part of the sentence that really concerns
you.)

When they are hungry. There's nothing you can do
about this one, try as you may. Your children will not be
hungry for you just because it's mealtime. On the contrary, they are often hungry between meals, like after
school and before dinner. You can't change that, so what
can you do about it?

YOUR JOB

You can concentrate on doing your part in that sentence—make foods available to your children when they are hungry. You can keep real foods around and offer your kids something they like and want, something their bodies can use well for fuel. Pleasure foods do not qualify because children's bodies do not need pleasure foods when their hunger signals a need for real fuel. That eliminates cookies, Twinkies, soda pop, cake, candy, and ice cream, to name a few of the favorite kids' pleasure foods. What's left for a between-meal snack, then?

BETWEEN-MEAL SNACK

Just the phrase limits the imagination: Between-meal snack. I have to take that one apart, too.

Between. It sounds so hurried and abrupt, something of an impulse, thoughtless and unimportant, squeezed in between other more important things.

Meal. This is such a misused and dangerous term that I have to discuss it separately, too. Generally, it refers to a considerable amount of food eaten at regular intervals. Meals are those other things that between-meal snacks are supposed to be squeezed in between.

Snack. This is another noncommittal word, like between, that suggests an unsubstantial, light food, usually not significant enough to be eaten at the table. A between-meal snack, then, is considered an unimportant, scanty amount of impulsively chosen food eaten on the run sometime before or after a legitimate meal. Why bother with it at all?

I prefer, for obvious reasons, to eliminate the phrase altogether. I will not refer to foods that are appropriate for hungry children or adults as between-meal snacks because they do not fit that description. I prefer the phrase, "real foods that children like."

REAL FOODS THAT CHILDREN LIKE

The biggest problem you will have with foods that fit into this category is that they sound like meal foods, not between-meal foods. They are real-meal foods, the best foods around. Real foods that children like include peanut-butter-and-jelly sandwiches (and all variations of bread, peanut butter, butter, and jelly), grilled cheese sandwiches, cheese and crackers, fruits of all kinds, all real-food leftovers, peanuts and other nuts with raisins or seeds, fried-egg and egg-salad sandwiches, toast and milk, hot or cold cereal, real juices, and English muffins. The list is endless. Make your own with your children's preferences in mind. It's easy. Just think of any real foods that your children like to eat. You don't have to be afraid to feed them real foods that they like when they are hungry. It's the most natural thing to do.

WHAT ABOUT SUPPER?

Won't all this after-school snacking (no, eating) spoil their supper? Whose supper? Their supper? No, your supper. Why should they have a supper when they aren't hungry? It doesn't make sense. But what about mealtime, eating with the rest of the family? What about it? What's so sacred about mealtime? Mostly your feelings. Being together as a family *is* sacred, and it is important, but who ever said you have to *eat* together to *be* together? You can still spend time together, but if a child isn't hungry then because he ate a sandwich and drank a glass of milk when he was starving after school, what's the big deal? Your feelings, if you're the one who fixed supper, but those feelings might be causing you and your family a lot of trouble. Maybe you should think about changing them, along with some other unhelpful mealtime routines.

THE SUPPER SCENE

Usually the worst time of the day for a family is just before supper. The reason is obvious. Everybody is starving. Consequently, everyone is also irritable, tense, tired, and impatient to eat. Children have been held off since they came home from school with a between meal snack. You already know how well and how long that probably kept them satisfied. Dad had a light lunch at noon because he's watching his weight and had to fight the five-o'clock traffic while he had a splitting low-blood-sugar headache. Mom had cottage cheese and fruit at noon, bouillon at three, black coffee at four, carrot sticks at four-thirty, and a violent outburst of anger at five. All the kid said was, "When's supper going to be ready? We're starved!" and she exploded.

HOW TO HELP

As you learn to get in touch with your own body's needs, likes, and patterns, and as you begin to satisfy your physical needs for fuel according to your body's signals, you will also be able to help other people in your home get in touch with their bodies. This is very different from trying to control others' eating habits. You are letting go of the controls and giving them back to their rightful bodies. Instead of feeding your children as if they were willful, ignorant infants, you can allow them to eat much more according to their own bodies' signals—what, when, and how much. Don't worry. As long as you provide lots of real foods that they like to eat, they will choose well.

WHAT'S IMPORTANT

As for mealtimes, try scheduling them more according to the general concensus of hunger instead of strictly by the clock. Perhaps a mini-meal after school with a slightly later supper would work. Dad, and Mom if she works away from home, too, could have hors d'oeuvres immediately when they get home. Little changes can save everyone a lot of strain. There may not be anything sacred about eating together every day, but there is definitely something sacred about being kind to each other.

CHAPTER 9
GETTING STARTED FOR GOOD:
WHAT TO DO,
WHAT TO EXPECT

HOW TO GET STARTED

The first step toward permanent thinness is to find out if you are on the Feast-or-Famine Cycle. This step will help you in several ways. You will become more aware of how your undereating has affected your overeating behavior. You will become familiar with the classic signs of Feast-or-Famine Cycle so you can be alert to these warning signals in the future. And you can stay clear of situations that provoke any of these old behaviors.

STEP #1: CHECK YOURSELF FOR SIGNS OF THE FEAST-OR-FAMINE CYCLE

There are six clues to the Feast-or-Famine Cycle experience. Check yourself for each one:

1. Binging or regular overeating.
2. Excessive hunger or symptoms of low blood sugar (see p. 119)

3. Cravings for pleasure foods (sweets and high-fat foods)
4. Eating without real hunger, especially at night
5. Special occasion overeating.
6. Fear and/or guilt about eating.

If you are having any or all of these symptoms, you are still caught in the Cycle of undereating and overeating.

But take heart and keep reading. You will be Cycle-free very soon! If you no longer have these symptoms because you have started eating anytime you're hungry, you are already making great progress. You have begun to break the vicious Cycle that causes your weight problem.

STEP #2: LIST HUNGER SIGNALS AND MIMICS

First, list all the ways your body "asks" for fuel: hunger, empty sensation, gurgling stomach, headache, dizziness, irritability, etc.

Second, check some other important influences on your eating behavior. Make a list of other eating triggers. Although excessive hunger (from undereating) is almost always the most important factor in overeating problems, other stressors are likely to mimic hunger and influence eating habits. These include fatigue, thirst, and tension from inactivity. There is always a good reason behind a binge or compulsive eating—needs. If the need is *not* actual physical hunger (and you will be better able to sort out your needs as you go along), then satisfy the real need.

STEP #3: ADJUST FOOD AVAILABILITY

Third, adjust the food availability in your environment. This is vital to your success. A good variety of high quality foods that you like must be available for you to eat any time your body sends a hunger signal. Pleasure foods must be eliminated from the environment, not because pleasure foods are bad, but because they are inappropriate for your body's new need to eliminate excess fat. Your goal now is to provide your body with an environment of optimal (best, most nearly perfect, highest quality) food availability. So, buy lots of delicious real foods and get rid of the junk—now!

STEP #4: EAT ACCORDING TO YOUR BODY SIGNALS

Once you have made real food readily available to your body, you can begin to eat according to your body's fuel-need signals. Learn to listen carefully to your body signals, especially hunger. Since your body's needs will change as your eating changes, be flexible, ready for changes in your body's fuel needs and signals. You'll probably be surprised at how often you're hungry and how much or little you want/need to eat. Whenever you get a fuel-need signal, trust your body by eating real foods you feel hungry for. Stop eating when you feel full.

Getting started is just that simple—four easy steps to permanent thinness!

- Check yourself for symptoms of the Cycle
- List hunger signals and other eating influences
- Adjust your Food Availability Factor
- Eat when you're hungry until you're not

WHAT YOU CAN EXPECT TO HAPPEN WHEN YOU GET OFF THE FEAST-OR-FAMINE CYCLE

First, you might gain. If you have recently been on a typical diet, and undereating or eating-avoidance were an important part of the program, you will need to gain weight by overeating. So, of course, you will overeat and gain weight—for a while. This will be your body's last feast, and it is necessary to end the Feast-or-Famine Cycle forever. (Everyone ends with a feast.)

This weight gain can be frightening for weight-conscious dieters, but they need to persist in faith and if possible get some genuine support for themselves during this time of transition.

How much do you gain, anyway? The amount of weight you gain during this period will depend on:

1. How much you lost on your recent diet.
2. How long and severe the diet (famine) was.
3. How well you begin to provide real food to meet your body's needs now.
4. Your overall diet history.
5. Your inherited sensitivity to food availability.

You may gain less than five pounds if your dieting has been minimal and you usually eat fairly regularly. But if you have been very hard on your body, going hungry often, perhaps with exercise, and the undereating/overeating Cycle has been very extreme, you will gain more than that.

You are likely to gain at least as much as you just lost by starving yourself. But you'll gain it back eventually anyway if you keep trying to diet. So what have you got to lose? A lot of weight, right? Let's move on to the losing part before everybody gets discouraged!

YOUR BODY IS CHANGING INSIDE

While your body is in this transition phase of getting off the Cycle, you will experience some odd changes. These changes in your body's hunger and eating interests herald the beginning of your weight loss. You will eat differently and develop a new, healthy relationship with food. This may go on for some time (three to 12 months) before you actually see weight loss according to the scale. But inside, it is happening, and you can take the following new experiences as proof of your body's new need to get slim.

PROOF THAT YOU BODY'S NEED FOR FAT IS DISAPPEARING

First, your hunger and appetite will "normalize".
1. Binging will stop.
2. Eating will shift to earlier in the day.
3. Night eating will diminish greatly.
4. Cravings will change to real foods.
5. Interest in pleasure foods will diminish dramatically.
6. Satisfaction point will become well defined. (You will know when you are full.)
7. Body signals will govern all eating behavior.

Second, your emotions will stabilize.
1. You will stop feeling guilty about eating.
2. You will become more relaxed in general.
3. You will feel more patient and less irritable.
4. You will begin to feel better about yourself.
5. You will be less and less concerned about and preoccupied with your diet.
6. You will have more emotional and physical energy.

Once your last feast has ended, your appetite has normalized, and your emotions have stabilized, your body will begin to burn its stored fat. This is it! You lose weight!
1. Your body adapts to your new eating patterns by gradually decreasing your appetite.
2. You respond to this change by eating less and/or lighter foods.
3. You naturally eat less food than you need to maintain your weight.
4. Your body burns stored fat to make up the difference.

5. You lose weight until your body reaches its ideal adapted weight in an environment of optimal food availability.
6. Your body maintains your newly adapted trim shape by the same means that led to your natural weight loss.
7. As long as you continue to eat well, you never gain unnecessary weight again.

Remember! Your body's ideal weight depends on the food availability of its environment—the type and amount of food you eat and when you eat it. The most adaptive weight for a person who provides her body with a good variety of high quality foods at all times is trim. This is what your body will need if you provide such an environment.

HOW LONG WILL IT TAKE TO LOSE THE WEIGHT ONCE YOU GET COMPLETELY OFF THE CYCLE?

This depends on several factors. The first five are up to you. The last two are your body's responsibility.

YOUR JOB

1. Quality of the foods you eat.
2. Variety and balance of the foods you eat.
3. How well you listen and respond to your body's fuel-need and other-need signals.
4. Avoidance of pleasure foods.
5. Managing the food availability in your environment.

YOUR BODY'S BUSINESS

1. How much excess weight your body has to lose.
2. Your body's unique adaptive potential.

Some bodies are more adaptable than others. They adjust to changes in the environment more readily than others. In the case of obesity, some are very efficient at fat storage, binge tolerance, and deprivation tolerance. Others do not have the flexibility to handle these stresses. This explains why some people never seem to have trouble with their weight. Their bodies simply won't take the abuse of unsatisfied hunger.

NO BODY LIKE YOURS

It follows, then, that your body's adjustment to this new availability of food will be unique. Try not to have rigid expectations, but be open to slow or faster adjustments, trusting your body to adapt perfectly in its own perfect time. You've been in control long enough. Now it's your body's turn. Let go.

QUESTION: HOW CAN YOU SPEED IT UP?

1. Make the very best variety of quality* foods available to your body as much as possible.
2. Avoid getting too hungry by planning ahead.
3. Carefully avoid pleasure and borderline foods (listed later in this chapter).
4. Review your eating habits once in a while to be sure you are satisfying your body's needs and troubleshoot problem areas.
5. Don't weight yourself.
6. Choose lighter foods and beverages for bedtime.
7. Get some genuine support.
8. Drink plenty of water every day (this is an essential ingredient in fat metabolism).

QUESTION: HOW CAN YOU SLOW IT DOWN?

1. Don't be overly concerned with the quality, variety, and overall availability of foods.
2. Let your body get excessively hungry on a regular basis.

*low-fat/low sugar

3. Rationalize frequent eating of pleasure and borderline foods.
4. Keep trying to control your eating at least some of the time.
5. Weigh yourself as often as possible.
6. When you are a little hungry at bedtime, eat something rich.
7. Avoid drinking extra water.

Now, back to the original question. *How long will it take?* Once you stop gaining, level off, and begin to finally lose, how long will it take to lose weight?

Answer: It will take, on the average, one month to lose two to six pounds, permanently. This does not mean that you will lose one or two pounds the first week. Remember, the first weeks you may be gaining, getting off the Cycle. But once you do start the *gradual* downward trend, you can safely expect your body to be able to handle a loss of between two and six pounds a month. It is possible in a given month, for you to lose more than that naturally (usually this represents intermittent diuresis during slow, steady weight loss). It is likewise possible for your body to give up less than two pounds in a given month, or to plateau at certain weights for weeks or even months.

If you lose weight faster, be sure you are not famining or going hungry to do it. Otherwise you will gain it back. If you lose less, fine. It's still permanent weight loss without hunger, and you will eventually lose whatever you have to lose to be thin. In my experience, it is often the more obese that lose faster while the moderate overweights seem to need more time. But there are no rules here!

CHANGING YOUR BIOCHEMICALS

All organisms adjust to changes in the environment by

various delicate communications systems. One of the most important involves biochemicals. Biochemicals are simply substances that perform biological duties. Vitamins and hormones are common biochemicals.

HAVES AND HAVE NOTS

Studies have shown that obese people have certain biochemicals in their blood that nonobese people do not have. I believe that the body produces these special obesity chemicals in response to dietary deficiencies. Of course, these deficiencies can be the result of true variations in food availability, but we do not normally suffer from such environmental variations. We do, however, suffer dietary deficiencies which the traditional quick-weight-loss diet imposes. Our bodies cannot discriminate between internal and external causes. All our bodies know is what they get, or don't get.

COURAGE TO CHANGE THE THINGS WE CAN

Changing your biochemicals is a matter of changing what your body gets, and you can control that. By eating well every day you can eliminate those obesity chemicals which I believe cause overeating and interest in fat-producing foods. If you give your body the good food it needs, you can help it normalize and adapt to this wonderfully plentiful land. We have so much delicious and healthful food. Isn't it about time you enjoyed some of it?

SEASONAL VARIATIONS IN WEIGHT

Seasonal fluctuations in weight for slim, healthy people are not uncommon. Many people expect to gain a little weight when the temperatures begin to drop. Often these extra pounds melt away in the spring and early summer without much effort. I have only observed northern North American climates, though. It might be less common where temperatures do not drop below freezing.

I believe this is a remnant of our bodies' abilities to use fat storage to adjust to the demands of different environments. It also reflects the important role that fat still plays in insulating us against the weather, an adaptive response to the stress of cold climates. But whether for warmth or food, the body does not make changes without a good reason. You can trust your body.

FOR THOSE WHO WATCH THEIR WEIGHT

If I never see a bathroom scale again as long as I live, by the time I die, I'll have saved a lot of time for more important things. If the idea of losing your little weight-guage frightens you, you are a true weight watcher.

Just like bird watchers, though, you can watch until the cows come home, but you will never have control over what you're watching. The closer you try to get to the birds, the more elusive they will be, not because they are not friendly or sociable, but because flying away at the approach of a human is a matter of survival. They are not judging motives. They need to stay alive.

It's the same with the body. It isn't concerned about how desperately you want to lose weight or how much you have already suffered trying to do so. It is physical. It cannot consider vain and lofty goals. Your body's first and most important job is to stay alive by the best possible means.

Modern Idolatry

The bathroom scale has become something of a god for the many weight-watching people of the world. Its blessing, showing a loss on a given day, can make the worst of circumstances easier to take. But its curse, the little needle moving upward, will cast a depressing shadow on the best of times.

In some ways, the invention of the scale was a sad discovery for human beings. Scales beget the bondage of pettiness, anxiety, and living by the letter of the law.

My advice? Throw it out today. It is not an asset to an ex-weight watcher who wants to become Naturally Thin.

INTRODUCTION TO FOOD CATEGORIES

Throughout the book I have referred to two basic kinds of food—real foods and pleasure foods. I have listed the foods which decidedly belong to these groups, and I have added one group in the middle. The in-between foods are called borderline foods because they have significant real foods in them but do not qualify as real foods because of high sugar or fat content. Sugar and fat, remember, are the main ingredients in pleasure foods.

QUALITY AND VARIETY COUNT

These food groupings are simple, general guidelines for choosing the highest quality foods. You can only eliminate the need for fat storage by eating a good variety of high quality foods according to your body's fuel-need (hunger) signals. The real-foods list is divided into the five traditional nutrient groups to help you check variety and balance in your diet. Variety ensures your overall nutrient balance, including vitamin and mineral intake.

You'll notice that the real-foods list is by far the longest and includes large food groups such as all fruits and all beef dishes. Your freedom to eat such a wide variety of foods and still gradually lose weight depends on your care in keeping your hunger well satisfied. Once your body recovers from the Feast-or-Famine Cycle, your appetite can comfortably decrease to a weight-reduction intake. When this happens, real foods will be the ones your body needs and consequently the ones you crave most.

Food preparation is influential in the quality of your diet because it can significantly affect the fat content of foods. Medical research has clearly shown that lowering saturated (especially animal) fat in the diet is beneficial in many ways. Also, fat calories are condensed (concentrated) and will fill you up in place of more necessary and healthful food varieties.

So fat intake definitely influences both the quality and variety of the diet. Your body will give up its fat stores more readily on a lower-fat, higher-quality food program. Fat calories are not as important as the detrimental effects fats have on the quality and variety of your diet.

FAT WILL SLOW YOU DOWN

Real foods can easily be turned into borderline foods. All you have to do is deep fry with breading or add heavy cream, cheese sauces, syrups, or fatty gravy and this will greatly slow down your body's need to burn up your fat stores. It may well stop you altogether if the fat content is high enough to destroy the quality and variety of your diet. A high-fat diet does not give your body the go-ahead to burn stored fuel. Instead, it sends the save-up-for-winter message. Since you know how your body responds to such a message, take care not to send it.

This does not mean that you can never fry anything or use butter, gravy, or sour cream as, say, vegetable condiments. A small amount of fat is important in a balanced diet, but you can get that small amount without adding it in. Just focus on eating well according to your body's fuel-need signals, with your appetite interests in mind. By the way, everyone, not just people with weight problems, should lower excess fats in their diet.

BORDERLINE FOODS ARE LOWER-QUALITY FOODS

Borderline foods are not particularly high-quality foods. If you can get along without them without suffering much, by all means do. The real foods are so much better for your body's purposes. This borderline list is just a guideline, again, and meant only to help you break the Feast-or-Famine Cycle as quickly as possible. If you get stuck for weeks and weeks, check this list, and try to eliminate these foods as best you can.

PLEASURE FOODS HAVE A PLACE

Pleasure foods are for any special occasion, not just the usual birthday, anniversary, holiday occasions. These foods are reserved for those rare times when your body sends strong signals for a pleasure food. No rules here, either, but you and I both know how much your body will actually need these foods once you are off the Cycle. So the signals will only occur naturally once in a while. Otherwise something's wrong in your diet. Check it out.

Don't panic about giving these foods up all of a sudden because, even though you probably have had overwhelming cravings for the items listed here while you were dieting, you will lose the powerful urge to eat these foods. Naturally, in order to stop needing and wanting these goodies, you must stay fed-up on real foods. Don't expect it to happen overnight, but after a few weeks of eating well, keeping your hunger satisfied on real foods, you will lose interest in pleasure foods. No kidding! Try it!

KEEP A *VARIETY* OF REAL FOODS AVAILABLE

One last word about variety in your diet. It is not necessary or desirable to try to eat a well-balanced meal each time you get hungry. It isn't practical, either. Your body needs dietary balance and variety over time. All food groups should be well represented every few days. Each group—dairy, fish/meat, grains/breads, and fruits/vegetables, can easily be covered if you keep these foods readily available and easy to prepare. You'll get hungry for different things, and eventually you'll find that your body is quite picky from meal to meal. You might have to think about fruits and vegetables a little more at first. Work them in. They're important!

REAL FOOD LIST

Guideline: Any food, any time you're hungry.

DAIRY

Milk**
Cheese—all types**
Cottage Cheese**
Plain Yogurt** (you can sweeten and add fruit)
Eggs
Cream**
Sour Cream**
Milk/Cream-based soups**

BREADS, GRAINS, CEREALS

Bread
Bagels, English muffins, etc.
Nuts and Seeds—all types
Unsweetened Cereals. Whole grain is better.
Oatmeal, Cream of Wheat, etc.
Whole-Wheat Pasta—all dishes
White Pasta—if you can't get or don't like whole wheat
Sandwiches—all types with real food fillings
Brown and Wild Rice

**lower fat percentages preferred

White Rice—brown is better
Dumplings, Stuffing—whole-wheat preferred
Peanut Butter
Whole-Wheat and Bran Muffins
French Toast

MEAT, POULTRY, SEAFOOD

Beef—lean cuts, all dishes
Chicken—all dishes
Fish—all dishes
Turkey, other Poultry—all dishes
Hamburger—extra lean, all dishes
Pork—lean cuts, all dishes
Shellfish—all dishes
Soups—all types
Stews—all types

FRUITS AND VEGETABLES

ALL Fruits—fresh preferred, canned, stewed
ALL Vegetables—fresh and lightly cooked preferred, canned
Vegetable-based Dishes—i.e. Oriental stir-fry, Chow Mein
Fruit Jams and Jellies—all types
Juices—all types 100% juice, unsweetened only
Salads—all types
Salad Dressings—all types
Soups—all types

FATS, SPREADS, CONDIMENTS

Peanut Butter
Cream Cheese—whipped or low-fat preferred
Margarine
Butter
Mayonnaise—fat-reduced preferred
Jams and Jellies

Gravy—fat skimmed
Mustard
Ketchup
Honey and Syrup
Veggie Dips

BORDERLINE FOOD LIST (REAL/PLEASURE FOODS)

Guideline: Once or twice a week, maximum

Munchies
Fast Foods
Sweet Rolls, pastries, etc.
Cocktails, Beer, Wine
Bacon, Sausage, Processed Meats (salami, bologna)
Pancakes, Waffles
Deep-Fried ANYTHING
Pudding, Custard, Sweetened Yogurt
Pre-sweetened Cereal
Punch, Regular Soda Pop, All Sugar-based Drinks
Casseroles with heavy-cream-sauce base
Lamb
Spareribs
Frozen Pot Pies
Pizza
Potato Chips, Taco Chips, etc.

PLEASURE FOOD LIST

Guideline: Once or twice a month and be fed-up!

Cakes, Frosting
Chocolate
Candy Bars
Candies
Cookies and Bars
Coffee Cakes

Fudge
Special Desserts—Betties, Cobblers, Strudel, etc.
Pies, Pastries
Ice Cream
Ices and Sherbets
Pastries
Sweet Toppings, Syrups

NOTES

CHAPTER 10
31-DAY PLAN FOR DEPROGRAMMING OBESITY

MIND POWER

Attitude has a tremendous effect on behavior. Attitude is largely determined by understanding or belief, and understanding comes from information or sometimes the lack of it. Some information is true and helpful in guiding adaptive, healthy attitudes and consequent behaviors. Some information is untrue or only partly true and is not helpful in these ways. In fact, it can be very destructive, as is the case of the traditional diet.

THE WHOLE TRUTH

The traditional quick-weight-loss diet's misinformation is that people are fat because they eat too much. This is really a half-truth, and the half which is missing is the key to understanding obesity. The other half of the truth about obesity is that people eat too much because they often eat too late, eat poorly, eat too little, or don't eat at all. Once people understand the whole truth about this modern plague, I believe their attitudes about obesity, whether their own or others', will change. This in turn will bring changes in eating behavior, which will gradually lead to healthy, adaptive changes in individual body weights.

THE TOY MAKER

In all our scientific advancement we have become like the young boy who, upon getting a curious and remarkable new toy, obstinately refuses to be shown how the toy is made and how it is supposed to work. In his false pride, carelessness, and stubborn resistance to this information, he unwittingly abuses its intricate parts and becomes angry when the toy is damaged and can no longer serve his selfish whims.

Perhaps the child did not want to learn because, being a bright child, he suspected that he would have to control his careless, destructive impulses to care for the special toy properly. Had he followed his intuition about the toy (seeing immediately that it was built with the highest skill and finest materials in the world), he might have learned, little by little, to understand the fascinating ways the toy could bring him joy.

If the child is lucky and the maker of the toy nearby (perhaps it is his own father), the maker would surely attempt to show the child how he is only hurting himself by his willful ignorance of the toy's design.

The maker, finding the child attentive and open, would then try to explain the special sensitivities of such a delightful machine. He might try to convince the boy that he gave him the toy in the first place because he loves him, and it makes him sad to see the toy he created destroyed, and the boy he loves so disappointed.

If he listens to the maker, the boy will learn more about the toy and eventually grow to understand it quite well. He will want to take care of the toy because he appreciates the skill and purpose of its maker. And he will see what an irreplaceable gift it is.

In time something special will happen. As the boy

grows in understanding, appreciation, and love for the toy which was intended for his pleasure, he will also grow in understanding, appreciation, and love for the toy maker. They will become very close, talking together about the toy a great deal. They will talk about many other things, too. The maker will share his wonderful creative ideas about everything, and the curious boy will learn to believe the toy maker and trust what he says, even before he understands completely. He knows that the maker is full of wisdom and love in his creating.

TRUST, FEAR, OBSTACLES

Having no choice in the matter, babies live in complete trust. They start life from an attitude of faith, if you will. As they are cared for and loved, according to their needs, that trust is reinforced as they grow.

When a trusting child experiences something in his life for the very first time, he has no confining expectation, just a curious openness. He might be a little afraid because he is unaware, but a child seldom resists a new experience because he is anxious. If he is reassured by loving parents or friends, he will usually take courage and meet up with life. He will thrill at a dare and laugh in relief that life is really fun, even when it's new and scary. And when he is disappointed or hurt, as every child inevitably is, he can forget about it fairly easily, being a child.

The grownup is often more afraid than curious or daring, because life has not been fun. It has been full of disappointment and fear. An old person, not old in age but old in fear, does not get excited about new experiences anymore. He doesn't believe in them. He is so afraid of life that his greatest hope is that nothing new will come along to frighten him.

Unlike children, he is afraid of death too, so there is no joy at either end. And being old, he has forgotten how to forget like the children. Those who are old in fear are very unhappy and very lonely.

Often overweight dieters, having suffered years of discouragement about their weight problems, have grown old in their thinking and feelings, too. They are afraid.

FEAR IS THE ONLY OBSTACLE

The biggest obstacle that I have encountered in counseling overweight people with the Adaptation Theory ideas is this: There are *no* obstacles. There is only freedom to eat. This is frightening to people who have grown old in their struggle with obesity, aged by the heavy anxiety of dieting every day and in every way possible. They fear they will eat all day. They fear they will want only pleasure foods. They fear they will gain and gain and never level off or begin to lose.

Most dieters are frightened as they embark on this new way of thinking and eating, but as they begin to understand, their faith grows.

FAITH OVERCOMES FEAR

Usually, because they finally understand why they are overweight, they have the strength of mind to begin to act on their faith. But they must take care to act slowly and thoughtfully, one moment at a time. They must not try to change everything at once because changes must happen gradually and naturally. There must be no artificial force exerted that causes pain, or the body will surely resist for survival's sake. And resistance meets resistance, beginning a vicious cycle.

Once the freedom is accepted, these brave people enter into the last season of feasting. They recognize the symptoms of this side of the Feast-or-Famine Cycle— some overeating, cravings for pleasure foods, eating for no apparent reason. But because they understand what their bodies are doing (making up for the famines be-

fore understanding came), the fear begins to leave, and
they begin to enjoy eating as it was meant to be enjoyed.
The last feast ends and the vicious Feast-or-Famine
Cycle ends with it.

The world is not unjustly divided into two types of
bodies—those who gain weight relentlessly and those
who never gain at all. Those who gain do so because of
their efforts to lose, because of their ignorance. Each
body is built much the same with the same potential for
adaptation to the many diverse environments on earth.
And all fall prey to the error in people's thinking about
things they did not create, being just part of the creation
and not the Creator.

After a period of feasting, which is the last significant
overeating these people will ever experience, their
appetites begin to change. They begin to lose the old
desire for sweet, fat, junky food. They do not *want* to eat
as much. They do not feel compelled or overwhelmed
when they are around pleasure foods. They stop overeating entirely, even on special occasions. Their eating
is generally the same from day to day, week to week.
They recognize their diminishing hunger, and they have
gradually turned into picky eaters.

The old cravings pass away, and behold, new cravings
come—urges for peanut butter on toast and milk, a
specific desire for eggs or soup or spaghetti. At the same
time they experience a decided distaste or apathy for
old favorites like candies, ice cream, potato chips, and
gooey desserts. When they do have something sweet,
they have what they want, a little something just for the
fun of the taste. And since that's all they really want (and
apparently all they need), that's what they have.

REAL JOY

The suffering stops, the anxiety, guilt, self-rejection,
and pain slowly go away, the fear of food and fatness

vanishes. And all the while their faith grows strong and hope replaces despair. There is real joy for these people who have been sad for so long.

INTRODUCTION TO THE 31-DAY PLAN FOR DEPROGRAMMING OBESITY

YOU'LL NEED SUPPORT

With guidance and the evidence that it worked and keeps working for others, you can break the Cycle faster than I did and start losing weight sooner, too. But you'll need help—every day for a while.

For your day-to-day guidance, I have condensed the principles of this eating-to-get-thin concept into a 31-Day Plan which you can follow as you progress. I made this day-by-day review because so many people I've counseled expressed a need for daily support and reminders of this new way of getting thin.

I call it the Plan for Deprogramming Obesity because we have been carefully indoctrinated with the idea that eating too much causes obesity, and it takes an effort similar to deprogramming a cultist to erase the false beliefs and replace them with the whole truth. Together with the food lists, these readings will help you deprogram the old diet attitudes and beliefs which are deeply ingrained into your thinking.

THREE-MONTH MINIMUM

You will probably need to use this plan in monthly cycles until your understanding of obesity is strong and you are well on your way to becoming a natural thin. Of course, you needn't use the readings in exact order once you get going, but daily use of the plan for three months is very helpful to your permanent success. You may find some specific readings especially useful and important for your particular problems. Mark these pages and review them more often. You can also write your own.

❖

DAY ONE
KEY THEME: FREEDOM
OWNING YOUR DIET

I am responsible for my own body. I make the decisions that affect my body for good or bad. I enjoy the benefits and suffer the consequences of choices I make that affect my body. I am the only one who can make the choices which will ultimately result in my body's permanent and natural slimness. I am the only one who knows my body's hunger and other-need signals. I am in control of the availability of food in my environment. I choose when, where, what, and how much I eat. Now I understand that these choices can lead to my becoming a normal, thin person. I choose to choose wisely.

"Self-trust is the first secret of success."

Ralph Waldo Emerson

Food for Thought: I have permission to eat well, every day.

DAY TWO
KEY THEME: FAITH
BELIEVING IN YOUR BODY

In an environment of high-quality, high-variety food availability, the normal, adaptive weight is nonobese or trim. There is no need for excessive fat. Obesity is therefore maladaptive in an environment where good food is always available and eaten according to the body's fuel-need signals. Your body is the product of generations of human beings whose survival has been ensured through adapting to various levels of food availability. Your body knows how to become slim. It has a built-in need to use up fat which is unnecessary for its survival. You can make that fat unnecessary by eating well every day. Your body will do the rest.

"Reactivate the dynamic quality of confidence based on the realistic fact that you have the knowledge and the ability to do what needs doing … You know how to do it competently."   Norman Vincent Peale

Food for Thought: Getting slim *is* natural.

DAY THREE
KEY THEME: HOPE
TAKING YOUR TIME

Think back to a year ago, two years perhaps. Does it really seem that long ago now? If you have been suffering from the Feast-or-Famine Cycle, you may think, Yes, it has been a long year. Waiting to lose weight has a way of dragging on and on and on, especially when it's uncomfortable, even painful. But one or two years *without the pain* is not too big a price to pay to be cured of a lifetime of obesity. I think it is the best bargain around.

"We need some imaginative stimulus, some not impossible ideal such as may shape vague hope, and transform it into effective desire, to carry us year after year … through the routine work which is so large a part of life."   Walter Pater

Food for Thought: Same time next year.

DAY FOUR
KEY THEME: SKILL
FOOD AVAILABILITY CHECK

Check your Food Availability Factor for home, workplace, leisure and travel/vacation. Count the foods you have on hand in lists A and B for each environment.

A. Real Foods (p.225)   B. Borderline/Pleasure
                                  Foods (p. 227)

__ High quality foods.   __Borderline foods.
__ High variety foods.   __Pleasure foods.
__ Foods I like
__ Foods I can eat raw.
__ Foods I can prepare fast.
__ Foods I know my body needs.

How many times yesterday did you get hungry without
real food available? ___

How many times yesterday did you substitute borderline or pleasure foods for real food needs? ___

If you listed less than two to any item in list A, fix it.

If you listed more than zero to either item in list B,
consider it.

If you listed more than zero to either question, think
about it. Get some understanding and make some
changes for today.

"Nothing can work damage to me except myself. The
harm that I sustain I carry about with me and never am
a real sufferer except by my own fault."

St. Bernard

Food for Thought: You'll eat what's available, so take
care!

DAY FIVE
KEY THEME: INSIGHT
UNDERSTANDING OBESITY

Not eating causes obesity—not eating well, not eating
enough, and not eating on time. The cure for obesity is

the reverse. Eating well, eating enough, and eating on time will gradually cause weight loss and ultimately lead to natural slimness.

The concept is simple enough for a child to understand, but it is not an easy thing to do. It requires much more than insight. In order to make this concept work for you, you must change. Inside and out, you must change your whole approach to your diet and your eating habits. Your new understanding will provide the ongoing motivation for change. And your new-found freedom from hunger will eliminate the tendency to go back to the old ways of eating and thinking.

"Very little is needed to make a happy life. It is all within yourself, in your way of thinking."

Marcus Aurelius

Food for Thought: *Not* eating causes obesity.

DAY SIX
KEY THEME: LOVE
COMPASSION FOR YOURSELF, OTHERS

Once you understand obesity, you'll begin to see how helpless people really are when they don't understand it. If you don't know what's wrong, how can you fix it? And as we all know, the traditional diet "cure" has ironically been the cause of obesity for many people besides you and me.

First, stop blaming yourself for getting fat.

Next, resolve to forgive yourself for gorging, binging, starving, and gaining. That should be fairly easy since your efforts were made in good faith as you attempted to solve your weight problem. You didn't understand, and you weren't really in control. So forget it.

Finally, think of all the people you've secretly judged

for their "poor self-control." Think of them now with understanding.

"It is surely better to pardon too much than to condemn too much."   George Eliot

Food for Thought: To understand is to pardon.

❖

DAY SEVEN
KEY THEME: DISCIPLINE
CRAVINGS AND HABITS

Remember the difference between normal willpower and abnormal or superhuman willpower? (See p. 42.) In order to effectively handle your sure-to-come cravings for borderline and pleasure foods, you need only be concerned with the normal type of willpower. Why? Because you will only let yourself get normally hungry.

You will avoid excess hunger like the plague it is. You will not starve yourself. Consequently, you will not need to binge to catch up. You will discover, as I did, that you really do possess a fair share of self-control, and you will gladly use it to choose your diet wisely.

The first step in breaking a habit is to think about it.

"I would have you consider your judgment [willpower] and your appetite [hunger] as you would two loved guests in your house. Surely you would not honour one guest above the other; for he who is more mindful of one loses the love and the faith of both."

Kahlil Gibran

Food for Thought: Normal hunger, normal willpower.

❖

DAY EIGHT
KEY THEME: FREEDOM
TRYING NEW THINGS

New things, new experiences, new ideas and new approaches to old things all have something besides their newness in common. They all usually get people to react. Some people react with fear and defense, others with interest and excitement. The same newness can evoke two extreme reactions in two different people. The difference is in the people.

The novel ideas in this book and every new experience that lies before you as a result of these ideas has the potential to enrich your life. How deep and enduring the effect is depends on you—how you choose to react and respond. Of course, how you respond depends on who you are. If you don't especially like yourself or your response patterns, you can change. Just decide who you *want* to be. Then decide how you *want* to react. And do it.

"The greatest discovery of my generation is that human beings can alter their lives by altering their attitudes of mind."

William James

Food for Thought: Change by trying new things.

DAY NINE
KEY THEME: FAITH
FUEL-NEED SIGNALS

What exactly are your individual fuel needs, anyway? Only your body knows for sure. Oh, your doctor or a nutritionist might give you a general idea of the fuel on which you could get along. But even their bodies know a lot more than they do about their individual fuel needs.

How can you find out more about these physiological needs and how to satisfy them? By listening carefully to your body's fuel-need signals.

Listen and think. Listen when your body is just whispering the signal. Don't wait until it has to scream. By then you will be very uncomfortable. Invite your body to tell you what it needs. Treat it like a friend, and it will become one. Is there anything you can get your body just now? Is there a quiet need you could help satisfy?

"It is the privilege of wisdom to listen."

O. W. Holmes

Food for Thought: Tune in to your body signals.

DAY TEN
KEY THEME: HOPE
PERMANENT WEIGHT LOSS

Once you have completed the last Feast-or-Famine Cycle (remember, you will end with a feast), you will begin a gradual, irregular descent on the scale. (Don't weight yourself if you can help it.) Some people seem to be able to lose steadily at a nice clip of about two to six pounds a month. Most of us are not that predictable.

Overall, though, we experience the same gradual descent in weight as we persist in eating well. Some bodies are more resistant to change, and the wait for that initial loss seems terribly long (up to 12 months), but it *does* come. And when it does, the losing will often speed up. Just wait. What else can you do? Want to go back to dieting?

"Faith is the assurance of things hoped for, the conviction of things not seen."

Hebrews 11:1 (author unknown)

Food for Thought: Permanent weight loss is slow.

DAY ELEVEN
KEY THEME: SKILL
BALANCE IN EATING

Review the introduction to food categories and the real foods list, pp. 179-184. Jot down on scrap paper what you ate yesterday. Don't labor over it and don't bother with amounts. You want to check balance, not calories. Now classify each food you ate into one of the four food groups in the real foods list (i.e. Dairy, Breads/Grains, etc.). Is any group completely missing? Any group over-represented? Are fresh fruits and fresh vegetables rare?

Start a shopping list to fill in the gaps. Keep balance in mind when you order a meal out. Put fresh fruits where you can see them at home and/or at the office. In the car carry portable foods you tend to miss. Be creative. There are a thousand ways to achieve balance and some very important rewards!

"Habit is a cable; we weave a thread of it everyday, and at last we cannot break it."

Horace Mann

Food for Thought: Quality and variety *plus* balance.

DAY TWELVE
KEY THEME: INSIGHT
NEEDING FAT

The main reason that people who diet the old way go crazy, binge, and crave all the wrong foods is their need for fat. They unknowingly create this physiological (not psychological) need by going hungry much of the time. The rest of the time on the diet, they are underfed and poorly nourished. Their need to maintain and/or store more excess fat dwells in their bodies in the form of special biochemicals. These chemicals evoke overeating (binging) and create a high interest in fat-producing foods. We are indeed "fearfully and wonderfully made," and we'd better seek to understand our bodies or we risk never becoming the best we can be.

"Nature imitates herself: A grain thrown into good ground brings forth fruit: a principle thrown into a good mind brings forth fruit. Everything is created and conducted by the same Master,—the root, the branch, the fruits,—the principles, the consequences."

Blaise Pascal

Food for Thought: Do I still need fat?

DAY THIRTEEN
KEY THEME: LOVE
SELF-ESTEEM AND BODY IMAGE

Obesity holds people back. It keeps them half-down all the time. It often prevents its victims from really believing in themselves. Obesity is a thief. It robs people of their self-esteem. This is why I so desperately sought a way out for myself. I was being held back. I was half-down, I wasn't able to believe in myself because I was fat. The fatness itself didn't really cripple me. How I felt about being fat did it.

This is true of just about every fat person everywhere. Don't be fooled. Nobody escapes the negative self-concept effects of obesity. Nobody is content with their fatness, not even the rich and famous.

There is a way out for you, too. It begins with understanding but quickly leads to how you feel about yourself and your body. As you make the right choices in the kitchen, choose your attitudes wisely, too.

"If you want things to be different, perhaps the answer is to become different yourself. Become a self-believer."

Norman Vincent Peale

Food for Thought: I accept me.

DAY FOURTEEN
KEY THEME: DISCIPLINE
PLEASURE FOOD

There is nothing wrong with pleasure foods. They don't cause obesity, and eliminating them, by itself, won't cure it either. Why list them? Why even mention pleasure foods if there's nothing wrong with them?

Pleasure foods are just fine for fun. The trouble lies with the dieter who misuses them for real-food purposes. There are two main reasons why they are misused. First, the dieter is overhungry and craves fat-producing pleasure foods because she needs fat. Second, all too often when hunger strikes, pleasure foods are available and real foods are not. That's it in a nutshell. Now go do something about it.

"A man full-fed refuses honey, but even bitter food tastes sweet to a hungry man."

Proverbs 27:7

Food for Thought: Real food for a real body.

DAY FIFTEEN
KEY THEME: FREEDOM
OTHER PEOPLE PRESSURES

It takes a great deal of self-assuredness to withstand

the critical eye (or voice) of another. There will be many difficult moments for the person who embarks on this program because of the general belief that fat people shouldn't eat very much, if at all. For some, this will be the hardest part of the program. These people have carefully avoided eating in front of anyone. They have become closet eaters. They are very sensitive to rejection and criticism and have a strong need to be accepted. Are you in this group? You will need courage.

"Whatever you do, you need courage. Whatever course you decide upon, there is always someone to tell you, you are wrong. There are always difficulties arising which tempt you to believe that your critics are right. To map out a course of action, and follow it to an end, requires some of the same courage which a soldier needs. Peace has its victories, but it takes brave men to win them."

Ralph Waldo Emerson

Food for Thought: I don't eat for other people.

DAY SIXTEEN
KEY THEME: FAITH
CLOTHES: STYLE AND COMFORT

You might be thinking, What do clothes have to do with faith? Good question.

I used to wear tight, uncomfortable clothes, especially pants, when I was dieting. I was using the tight clothes to frighten myself into realizing (as often as possible) just how fat I was getting. This would, I imagined, curtail my eating. And also I was punishing my body for its willful gluttony. Somehow, if I was in pain, I felt less guilty. So much for the psychological aspects of obesity.

The faith part comes in when you understand why you

are still fat and, further, how you can finally become slim. You realize that discomfort will only work against you. You see that your body is not to blame and needn't be punished. So you find the most attractive and comfortable outfit you can, and you wear it in good faith.

"In nature there are neither rewards nor punishments—there are consequences."

Robert G. Ingersoll

Food for Thought: I can look and feel better *now*.

DAY SEVENTEEN
KEY THEME: HOPE
PLATEAUS/WAITING

One of the goals of this program is to distract the chronic dieter. A major side effect of traditional dieting is a terrible preoccupation with eating and weight, do's and don'ts. This adds to the dieter's defeat because, coupled with chronic hunger, waiting and watching for something to happen creates a restlessness and impatience. "I'm suffering, I'm struggling, I'm following all the rules. C'mon, where's my reward?"

The rewards of this program are immediate although the weight loss is not. (Review pp. 172-174 if you are unsure about this.) For me the next best thing to getting thin was the freedom to think about other things, even while I was still losing! I let my body make the choices and do the work part of my diet. And I can concentrate on other, more important things.

"The secret of patience is doing something else in the meanwhile."

Apples of Gold

Food for Thought: Am I distracted?

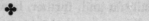

DAY EIGHTEEN
KEY THEME: SKILL
HUNGER IN DISGUISE

You are learning so much about your body these first few weeks! Perhaps you've been surprised a few times—when you get hungry, what you get hungry for, how much, how little you want or need to eat. It takes a considerable amount of trust in your body to keep on satisfying its fuel-need signals. But remember, as you satisfy it, its needs will change. Your body will need the same thing you need—to be slim.

If you are uncertain about a signal your body sends, ask yourself, Does any real food sound appealing? Does food suddenly look good to me? Would I probably feel better if I ate something? If you answer yes to any one question, try eating. You will soon discover whether or not you got the signal right.

"In today's thin world, our best chance is for the facts about fat to replace the myths about obesity."
        from "Fat Chance in a Thin World" *NOVA* Program
                                                    #1007

Food for Thought: When in doubt, try eating.

DAY NINETEEN
KEY THEME: INSIGHT
FATIGUE AND OTHER APPETITES

What about the times (and they will come) when you feel hungry but you honestly don't feel like eating? (This is quite a switch from the common dieter complaint of wanting to eat without feeling hungry!)

Don't eat if you don't feel like it, of course. But never

wander far from real food because your fuel-need could appear very quickly. Once you are off the Feast-or-Famine Cycle, your body will not tolerate unsatisfied hunger for very long. This intolerance is a good sign. Your body is adapting to a new environment of optimal food availability. It doesn't have to take the abuse of starvation anymore. Why should it?

Sometimes you may feel hungry when you have another physical need. Perhaps you are overtired or nervous or dehydrated. This is not uncommon, but it is easy to handle. As long as you keep your body well fed, there's no harm in mistaking your body's need for rest, etc., with its need for food. Gradually, you'll get better at knowing your body's signals and satisfying them.

"How can you come to know yourself? Never by thinking, always by doing."

Johann Wolfgang von Goethe

Food for Thought: Meet the right need.

DAY TWENTY
KEY THEME: LOVE
TAKING CARE OF YOURSELF—AN INVENTORY

Are you a martyr? Are you a victim? Are you waiting for someone to come along and rescue you from the sweat and strain of life? Are you into silent self-pity? Are you secretly proud of your habit of self-degradation? Do you have an exaggerated need for attention? Do you play the "Ain't-It-Awful Game" to get that attention? Are you usually prepared for the worst or are you getting ready for something good to happen?

Are you taking care of yourself, or are you trying to take care of everyone else in hopes that someone will notice your sacrificial spirit and take care of you? Are you as nice to yourself as you are to a good neighbor? Did you know that (besides God) you are the only one who can meet your needs and change your life in any significant way? Are you ready to succeed—or are you terrified that you might?

"I'm important to me! ... I mean much more to me than I mean to anybody I ever knew!"

The Unsinkable Molly Brown

Food for Thought: I am getting ready for success.

DAY TWENTY-ONE
KEY THEME: DISCIPLINE
EMOTIONAL EATING

There is some comfort in eating, but there is no comfort in being fat. Don't forget that. There are comforts in other activities as well, and I urge you to investigate them for your personal use.

Comforting activities can be directed toward others or toward ourselves: talking with a friend, helping someone, going for a walk, writing a letter, reading a good book.

Remind yourself today that so-called emotionally-inspired eating is intimately related to the Feast-or-Famine Cycle. (See pp. 85-90.) Getting off the Cycle should curtail the "refrigerator response" significantly, but habit may also play a role. So, if you find yourself in the kitchen asking yourself what you're hungry for and the answer is love, that's what you should have. It's up to you to get or give some.

"Great battles are really won before they are actually fought. To control our passions we must govern our habits, and keep watch over ourselves in the small details of everyday life."

Sir John Lubbock

Food for Thought: Food is physical fuel and not for feelings.

❖

DAY TWENTY-TWO
KEY THEME: FREEDOM
EATING OUT

I usually eat some real food just before going out to eat so I'll be comfortable enough to enjoy myself and alert enough to order intelligently. I used to save up my appetite for a meal away from home so I could eat without feeling too guilty.

That was a bad plan. At a restaurant, it always takes longer to actually get the food than you expect. So, if you're quite hungry when you go out, you'll likely be extremely hungry or starving by the time you're able to eat. Also, it is hard enough to order from a menu full of delicious meals when you are only slightly hungry. It's worse when you are starving. When you do get the food, it takes great restraint to savor and enjoy it because your blood sugar is at a critical low. The natural thing to do is gobble it up as fast as possible. But that tends to take some of the joy out of the experience. My advice is, dine early and eat before you go.

"It gives great glory to God for a person to live in this world using and appreciating the good things of life without care, without anxiety, and without inordinate passion."

Thomas Merton

Food for Thought: Enjoy the *whole* experience.

❖

DAY TWENTY-THREE
KEY THEME: FAITH
SICKNESS/STRESS

Ralph Waldo Emerson wrote, "First, be a good animal." Now this quotation might puzzle you at first, but think about it. No one advises animals in the wild which they should feed, a fever or a cold. So how do the animals know what to do when they are sick or under stress (danger)? They know by their bodies' signals, and they instinctively follow them. Hunger sends them hunting for food. Nausea demands a fast. Thirst is an invitation to drink. Its absence is a signal to stop. It is not complicated. Maybe that's why we humans have such trouble with it.

"Studies with animals have found that obesity is not a naturally occurring phenomenon."
from "Fat Chance in a Thin World" *NOVA* Program #1007
Food for Thought: Your body knows what it needs.

DAY TWENTY-FOUR
KEY THEME: HOPE
GETTING SUPPORT

You will probably need at least one other person to help you in this unconventional weight-loss program. Even if you don't feel a need for such a person, it's a good idea to find someone to talk with anyway. It is best if that person has read the book and shares a weight problem. (If your supporter hasn't read the book, get one for him or her to read.) Then you automatically have much in common.

If you can organize a group, however small, so much the better. Regular, informal meetings for sharing and

eviewing the principles of understanding obesity will
eep you going when changes are slow, especially at the
eginning. You'll also get a chance to help and encour-
ge others.

"Thou therefore which teachest another, teachest
ou not thyself?"   St. Paul
"No man is wise enough by himself."   Plautus
Food for Thought: I need supportive others.

DAY TWENTY-FIVE
KEY THEME: SKILL
RECOGNIZING THE FEAST-OR-FAMINE CYCLE

There are five main checkpoints that will indicate
whether or not you are on the Feast-or-Famine Cycle.
Any one of these factors can indicate a danger spot in
our diet. Once you are completely off the Cycle, you
hould be consistently free of these symptoms:

1. binging
2. excessive hunger
3. cravings for pleasure foods
4. urge to eat without hunger
5. special-occasion overeating

If you still have some of these problems, review Chap-
r 9. If you are completely symptom free (or nearly so),
ongratulations! You're on your way to becoming natu-
ally thin.

"Obese people, [dieters], one and all, described feel-
ng out of control during binges."   Author
"The worst day of my life was the day I found myself
ut of control."   Shirley McCullough, dieter
Food for Thought: Off the Cycle, in control.

DAY TWENTY-SIX
KEY THEME: INSIGHT
SWEETS

Sugar and sweet treats have such a bad name in our country today. Recently we've "discovered" that sweets are not only responsible for obesity but for a host of other major ailments as well. In fact, an entire best-selling book has been dedicated to the damnation of sweets and sugars.

I personally do not give sugar and her pleasure foods that much credit. It is clear to me that they don't cause obesity, and I'm not at all convinced that they, by themselves, cause much else, either. I'd have to blame the traditional quick-weight loss diet for many more nutrition-related diseases and disorders than sugar could ever cause.

I have already spent enough time in this book talking about the very minor role that sweets might appropriately play in the diet of a natural thin. (Naturally thin people seldom even have an opinion on the subject.) You must know the major part they have played in your feasts (binges). I trust that you've put it all together by now, and most likely you have some strong ideas of your own.

"Overweight is seldom just desserts."

Food for Thought: Real food is good for the sweet tooth.

DAY TWENTY-SEVEN
KEY THEME: LOVE
BEFRIENDING YOUR BODY

It is important that you make friends with your body before you get thin. The reason is simple. As friends, you and your body can get thin together. As enemies, neither of you will get there because of the sensitive lines of communication between your body and you.

If you dislike or even hate someone at the outset of a conversation, how much understanding ar you likely to achieve? How much cooperation? How much compromise? On the other hand, if you talk with a trusted friend, someone you love and respect, there will certainly be more understanding and cooperation between you.

Your body needs to be understood. It needs your help in its attempt to adapt healthfully to its environment. If you love it and respect its needs, your body will repay you with a wonderful gift. It will become naturally thin.

"For without words, in friendship, all thoughts, all desires, all expectations are born and shared, with joy that is unacclaimed."

Kahlil Gibran

Food for Thought: Your body is your friend indeed.

DAY TWENTY-EIGHT
KEY THEME: DISCIPLINE
EXERCISE

Exercise is said to be the component that can make or break the success of a diet program. It is true that regular exercise on the part of a dieter reflects to some extent her degree of commitment to getting into shape. But I disagree that exercise, by itself, determines whether or not a person wins at losing.

Certainly, regular physical activity has many health benefits. The question for you is not whether to exercise, but how to fit the best form of exercise into your lifestyle. I have made some suggestions in Chapter 7.

I've added a few ideas here to illustrate what I mean by fitting exercise into your lifestyle:

1. Buy a two-story or split-level house. (Bravo! if you already have one.)
2. Get a large dog.
3. Have a baby. (This is not the best reason to have one!)
4. Invest in some quality sports equipment.
5. Have a TV moratorium three days a week.
6. Plant a garden.

"I'm ... what's known as an athletic fat person."

Ray Goldsmith

"Fat Chance in a Thin World" *NOVA* Program #1007

Food for Thought: I can easily fit physical activity into my life.

DAY TWENTY-NINE
KEY THEME: FREEDOM
FORGETTING THE SCALE

Some dieters don't weight themselves. They're afraid to. Because they feel (and are) so out of control, they figure those numbers probably are, too. The negative experiences they have had all their dieting lives have conditioned them to avoid standing on the scale. For some, it is almost a phobia.

Most dieters are just the opposite. They weight themselves compulsively, even many times a day. They want to know, to be reassured, to feel more in control of their weight. This extreme is also fear motivated.

Once you turn your diet controls over to your body, you will need neither escape nor reassurance from the scale. You will know, as you provide plenty of good food for your body each day, that in time, you will be the perfect weight for you.

"I'm not overweight, I'm undertall."   Garfield

Food for Thought: Getting thin isn't a numbers game.

DAY THIRTY
KEY THEME: FAITH
LETTING GO

I hope by now that you're getting on nicely with the rest of your life. Stay busy! Be involved! Do new things! There is so much more to your life than your physical shape. And as you grow thinner naturally, you will discover that more of your real self will be free to emerge. You may even be surprised at the new you! Frankly, I am a better person since I stopped dieting and became thin. I suspect that you will be, too.

"Therefore I bid you put away anxious thoughts about food and drink to keep you alive, and clothes to cover your body. Surely life is more than food, the body more than clothes."

Jesus

Food for Thought: I'm getting better—all of me.

DAY THIRTY-ONE
KEY THEME: HOPE
IMAGING SUCCESS

There is a term used in psychology which I love. It is Creative Anticipation, and it refers to the fact that what you deeply expect to happen usually does. Whether or not you believe this does not alter its profound reality.

The power in this truth lies in the fact that our beliefs affect our behaviors. And our behaviors (including our choices) certainly influence what happens to us, what course our life takes.

So fill your thoughts with images of what you want to be and what you hope to accomplish. Chase the doubt and fear away. Be strong in your vision. Hold your ideal life firmly in your mind and never, never let it go.

"Because a thing seems difficult for you, do not think it is impossible for anyone to accomplish. But whatever is possible for another, believe that you, too, are capable of it."

Marcus Aurelius

Food for Thought: I can do it, too!

APPENDIX
OF CASE HISTORIES

I have selected six case histories to illustrate individual experiences with the process of becoming naturally thin. The people (and one cat) described here are real. Their names have not been changed. The details of their stories are accurately recorded so that readers can better understand how the recovery process works and how long it takes in various cases.

CASE #1 MARY ANN

Prerecovery statistics: Mary Ann, age 24, female

Weight: 135-160 unstable

diet history: 10 years

occupation: businesswoman

diet: eating-avoidance attempts to lose weight, undereating for two week periods followed by over-eating/binging and weight gain often exceeding starting weight, skips breakfast, low-calorie meals

cycle symptoms: preoccupation with weight and diet, chronic hunger later in day, absence of morning hunger, binging, overeating without perception of hunger, wide weight fluctuations, continuous resolutions to lose 30 pounds

motive for recovery: sick and tired of dieting unsuccessfully and feeling miserable about body-
weight
predisposition to obesity: mild to moderate (mild to
moderate obesity in siblings and parents)*

Mary Ann was really ready for the Anti-Diet at age 24.
She'd been dieting off and on for ten years even though
she knew it actually caused her to gain weight in the
long run. She didn't have any other options until I told
her about becoming naturally thin.

Ever since she was a freshman in high school, Mary
Ann had been trying to control her weight by not eating. Her sisters and parents were fighting the same
battle the same way. She was not a successful dieter, she
admits, because as soon as she tried to eat less, she became so hungry and preoccupied with food that she
always overate and gained weight. She understood the
link between dieting and overeating immediately when
I explained it to her. She'd experienced it in her own
life for years.

I spent about twenty minutes telling Mary Ann about
becoming naturally thin by eating more. She lived in a
different city from me, and the book was not available.
She had no support from anyone anywhere, and I didn't
hear from her for several years. I didn't know whether it
was possible for her to recover under these circumstances. Most people need a lot of encouragement and
support.

Mary Ann was so tired of dieting and going hungry
that the Anti-Diet was music to her ears. She went home
and started "doing it," as she puts it, which meant forgetting about dieting, eating real food whenever she got
hungry, and stopping when she was full. She began los-

*predisposition to obesity is generally higher in females

ing weight almost immediately! In fact, she lost weight so fast and so effortlessly that she went to her doctor convinced she was sick! Her doctor assured her that she was perfectly healthy, and she began to enjoy becoming naturally thin.

As a professional salesperson, Mary Ann worked at her office or met clients at their offices or in restaurants. She had to make some adjustments at work in order to keep real food available there. And she did, consistently meeting her hunger signals fast and with quality food during her busy workdays.

Mary Ann continued to lose for about six months although she didn't weigh herself (as I had recommended). When she did finally check her weight, she felt she had leveled off at normal thin, and she had lost a total of about 25 or 30 pounds. Her weight at that point was—naturally—right in the middle of the optimum range for a woman her height and frame.

Mary Ann has married and had a baby since then. She gained a healthy thirty pounds during the pregnancy. Although she felt plump and out of shape after the birth, she resisted the temptation to diet and ate her way down to her prepregnancy weight in just two months!

Mary Ann says that the greatest thing about being naturally thin, after actually being thin, is never having to worry about your weight. She spent so many years overweight and determined to lose weight that the thought strikes her every New Year's Eve—she doesn't have to resolve to lose thirty pounds! Mary Ann doesn't have thirty pounds to lose! She's busy resolving to do other important things and enjoying the wonderful freedom of being naturally thin.

Post recovery statistics: Mary Ann, age 29
weight: 128 stable
recovery history: five years at ideal weight

occupation: businesswoman, domestic engineer (mother/homemaker)

diet: eats about five times a day according to hunger, always eats breakfast, light meals frequently when on a schedule

cycle symptoms: none

recovery status: cured

effect of mild to moderate predisposition to obesity: conversion to naturally thin very rapid and without initial post-diet weight gain *in spite of* apparent familial tendency and female sensitivity to obesity. Every body is different.

❖

CASE #2 CAROL

Prerecovery statistics: Carol, age 28, female

weight: 175

diet history: 13 years

occupation: university student, domestic engineer

diet: rigid eating schedule to control appetite, low-calorie foods followed by junk-food binges, eating all meals but avoiding any between-meal eating

cycle symptoms: chronically undersatisfied hunger, emotional tension and irritability from hunger, weight fluctuations, preoccupation with dieting and weight, inability to lose weight by strict dieting

motive for recovery: fear of staying fat forever, unable to lose weight at all by conventional dieting methods, sick of chronic hunger and fatigue, tired of weight preoccupation

predisposition to obesity: High (less than two years postpartum, parents and siblings with moderate to serious weight problems)

Carol began the Feast-or-Famine Cycle with a medically imposed famine. She had her tonsils removed when she was twelve and couldn't eat much for several weeks. Although she was not overweight before the surgery, Carol recalls that she was fairly chubby by the time she was thirteen. She made some vague attempts at dieting and remembers binging on candy after school but had no success at losing weight until she was about sixteen. Then, almost magically and without effort, she grew thin.

Feeling she was not thin enough, Carol tried various diets again when she turned eighteen. She was unable to eat normally when she got braces during college and experienced binging and weight fluctuations again then. Naturally, she dieted before her wedding and then gained weight the following year. She had just started a new diet with renewed determination when she found out she was pregnant with her first baby.

Everybody "knows" that babies have a way of ruining a girl's figure for good. And when a woman's body conceives immediately after a month-long famine, that body needs fat and needs it badly. Remember, two lives depend on it now! So Carol gained weight quickly. Fifty pounds later she delivered a healthy baby boy.

She lost thirty pounds following delivery without much effort but plateaued at 175—not exactly svelte! She might have gradually continued to lose if she'd given her body enough time, but impatience caused Carol to try her old standby diet again. This time it was different. She couldn't lose anymore. No matter how little she ate, her extra pounds wouldn't budge.

Carol was afraid to try the Anti-Diet. The initial weight gain I had told her about scared her because she had been dieting strenuously. She knew she'd have to overeat and gain before she leveled off and started losing. The idea of going *up* from 175 was too much. She told me she had to try dieting one more time before she could give up on it completely.

So she tried her last diet. But she could not lose a pound and felt absolutely miserable. Hopelessly, she agreed to try eating more. Her prediction had been right on target. She gained about ten pounds during the first three months of Anti-Diet eating. She leveled off and then lost those ten pounds during the following two months. She was back where she started and hoped to keep going down. It didn't happen. She plateaued for nearly six months!

Even though her weight wasn't changing during this plateau, Carol's eating changed dramatically. Her cravings for sweets and junk food disappeared. She ate often, especially in the morning. She became ravenous at times but often found that this serious hunger was easily satisfied by a rather modest portion of real food. Her hunger and fuel-full signals became distinct. Eating became a completely internal, body-controlled behavior. She was eating like a naturally thin person, but she was still quite overweight.

Then, just to complicate her situation, she became pregnant with her second baby. If she was frightened before she started the Anti-Diet, she was panic stricken now! She was terrified of gaining another fifty pounds, the amount she had gained during her first pregnancy. I was confident that she wouldn't gain that much weight because she no longer physically needed the extra fat, but I had a tough time convincing her.

Convinced or not, Carol continued to eat freely. To her utter amazement, she began to gradually *lose weight* during the first four months of her pregnancy! She was *not trying* to lose weight by dieting or restricting her food and fluid intake. She was eating all the real food she wanted whenever she got hungry and only stopped when she was completely satisfied. (Pregnant women should not try to lose weight.)

Carol's doctor expressed concern about her weight loss so she brought her husband to the doctor to vouch for her eating habits. He assured the doctor that she was eating plenty and often!

Carol lost four pounds that first four months while her baby developed on schedule. That may not astound you, but compared to her more-than twenty-pound gain in the first four months of her earlier pregnancy, she already netted a twenty-four pound deficit! This encouraged her greatly.

Gradually, Carol began to gain after that but stayed far behind the fifty-pound gain of her first pregnancy. By her seventh month she had gained only fourteen pounds. When you consider the weight of a normal baby, plus placenta, plus extra fluid, Carol's own body was still getting thinner—and it showed! Her face, arms, and legs appeared more and more slender and clothes fit looser, too. Carol was becoming naturally thin right in the middle of a pregnancy!

Carol's story is not over. She now has two sons, ages one and three. She has lost over 40 pounds since her last baby was born. That puts her about 10 pounds below her starting point on the Anti-Diet. Her weight loss has been slow (just under three pounds a month), but steady. She keeps shrinking inside her jeans and has to buy a smaller size each time she replaces an old pair.

Carol has been discouraged at times but has persisted in her determination to be free to eat and thin too. Although not at her ideal weight yet, Carol is busy improving the quality of her *whole* life. She is in an exercise class that she enjoys, the first one in her life. She is working on her communication skills and her marriage. She is challenging herself in many important ways, as an individual, and as a wife, mother, daughter, sister and friend. Carol's hunger and eating have taken a quiet little place in her new life. For Carol, becoming naturally thin is just a matter of time.

Post recovery statistics: Carol, age 31
weight: 166
recovery history: two and one-half years off Feast-or-
   Famine Cycle, loss to ideal weight complicated by
   pregnancy
occupation: university student, domestic engineer
diet: two or three meals early in the day, real food
   anytime hunger strikes, no sweets, plenty of fluids,
   lighter meals at night, rare junk food, no overeating—ever
cycle symptoms: none
recovery status: in process of recovering ideal body-
   weight, excellent prognosis for cure
effect of high predisposition to obesity: nearly one
   year off Feast-or-Famine Cycle to begin true weight
   loss, weight gain of ten pounds getting off Feast-or-
   Famine Cycle, six month plateau preceeding real
   fat/weight loss

❖

CASE #3, TERRY

Prerecovery statistics: Terry, age 28, male
weight: 185-189, gradually increasing since college
diet history: no formal attempts to control weight
occupation: professional sales
diet: usually skipped breakfast or had juice and coffee
   only (not hungry in the morning), regular lunch
   by afternoon, no snacks, big supper with second
   helpings
cycle symptoms: night eating majority of daily
   calories, little or no morning hunger, getting overly
   hungry frequently during the day, overeating and
   eating seconds without perceptible hunger, gradual weight gain

    motive for recovery: concern about weight gain since
       college, clothes too tight, desire to reverse the gain-
       ing trend before serious weight problem
    predisposition to obesity: low (no significant obesity
       in parents or siblings)

Terry gave little thought to his weight until about five years after college. Gradually, he became aware that his waist was slowly expanding. As a professional salesman, Terry spent most of his workdays and some evenings seeing clients at various locations around town. He didn't think about his diet much until his wife, Carol (case #2), asked me to teach her the Anti-Diet.

Terry got most of the concepts second hand through Carol's experience of getting off the Feast-or-Famine Cycle. He said the thing that struck him about the approach was that he could (and should!) go ahead and eat when he got hungry and stop trying to not eat to lose weight. Even though Terry wasn't making a conscious effort to diet, he was still avoiding eating in an attempt to control his gradual weight gain. This put him on the Cycle, of course, which accounts for the weight gain he was unconsciously trying to fix.

The first thing Terry did to change his eating was to avoid second helpings after supper. He learned from Carol that nighttime overeating is largely responsible for keeping the fat going for people on the Cycle. So, he began pushing himself away from the table after a normal, medium-sized meal. The fact that he could push himself away from the table at night tells me that he was not seriously underfed. (As we know, people who diet strenuously often cannot stop eating by simply deciding to stop.)

This change caused Terry to begin to experience morning hunger for the first time in years. He began to eat immediately when he felt hungry in the morning—

usually by 9:00, about an hour or two after he got up. After he was on this breakfast schedule for a while, Terry noticed that he couldn't skip breakfast anymore. He got too hungry and weak. His body began to demand fuel early in the day. His night eating continued to be moderate without much effort.

Over a period of three or four months, Terry lost between fifteen and twenty pounds. He made a serious effort to change his eating patterns to better meet his body's needs, but he did not go hungry. He eliminated overeating at night by choice and added necessary calories and nutrients early in the day by his body's natural adjustment and demand. The fat loss that resulted was a natural physiological adaptation to the improved availability of food in the environment.

Terry is a good example of a person who gets on the Feast-or-Famine Cycle simply by eating late every day. Although his weight problem was not serious, Terry couldn't reverse the trend without understanding what was happening to his body as a result of his negligent eating habits and unconscious attempts to control his weight by eating avoidance.

Post recovery statistics: Terry, age 34
weight: 169-174
recovery history: over two years at ideal weight
occupation: professional salesman
diet: breakfast by 9 a.m., if misses breakfast, very early
    lunch by 11 a.m., always orders food if hungry
    when meeting client at a restaurant, keeps hunger
    in mind when planning schedule, no large meals,
    consistently more eating in the morning/less at
    night
cycle symptoms: none
recovery status: cured
effect of low predisposition to obesity: off Feast-or-

Famine Cycle in about a week, no weight gain getting off Cycle, very fast natural weight loss once off Cycle

♣

CASE #4, KAREN

Prerecovery statistics: Karen, age 30, female, postpartum

weight: 132-145 unstable

diet history: twenty years

occupation: domestic engineer, musician

diet: low calorie, eating avoidance, exercise to burn calories, eating out of control on weekends and evenings, binging on sweets (brownies, chocolates, fudge)

cycle symptoms: starving, skipping meals (especially breakfast and lunch), binging and overeating, weight fluctuations, preoccupation with dieting and weight, poor body image (at "ideal" weight)

motive for recovery: very tired of the hopeless cycle and all the pain of going hungry and being out of control, willing to let go and gain weight temporarily for the long-term goal of diet-free lifestyle

predisposition to obesity: high, less than two years postpartum and mother and sisters with serious obesity

Karen started worrying about her weight and trying to control her appetite even before she was in high school. Since her mother was very overweight and always dieting, Karen knew without being told that she'd better starve herself if she wanted to stay thin. And she did with fair success—if you call fluctuating between 132 and 145 pounds on 600 calories a day a success. Even within this weight range, which is considered slightly underweight to normal for her height and bone size, Karen hated her body proportions. She was chronically hungry and pre-occupied with dieting and weight loss.

Of course, Karen didn't eat 600 calories every day. She binged in the evenings and especially went out of control on the weekends. She devoured pans of brownies and fudge and ate big bags of M & Ms candies when her body overpowered her willpower. Her M.O. was famine during the week as best you can, feast all weekend. By the time she'd had three babies in four years, starving and exercising herself back to 145 between pregnancies, Karen was sick and tired of the Cycle. She was ready for the Anti-Diet.

Karen understood the Anti-Diet concepts instantly and stopped dieting. She knew she'd gain weight but was hopeful that eventually she could live a normal diet-free life. Almost immediately, she became pregnant with her fourth baby in five years. Naturally, this complicated the situation but Karen persisted in letting her body control her eating. She gained more weight than a nor-mal, nondieting mom because all those years of crazy dieting had taught her body to need extra fat. She gained 65 pounds in the pregnancy but was learning how to tune into her body signals during that time. She ate high-quality, real food most of the time.

Following a normal delivery of a big, healthy baby boy, Karen lost 15 pounds during the next year by eating freely according to her body signals. She grew restless to lose more and faster, but she persisted in eating real food on time and never going hungry.

Karen plateaued another whole year. She was under huge personal stress during this time, which she thinks contributed to her weight maintenance. Perhaps her body wasn't willing to change with all the changes going on in her environment—four children under five-years-old at home and a divorce in the works. Still, as Karen worked at accepting herself and her body, she met the daily challenges of life.

Finally, Karen felt it was time to give her body a boost. She decided to cut way down on fats since this is the best way to improve quality. (See "How Can You Speed It Up?" on p. 175.) She eliminated most dairy products (high fat ones) and limited red meats to once a week since they also have higher fat content. She ate unlimited amounts of chicken (no skin, to lessen fat) and fish (no butter, oil, or sauces), fruits, vegetables, pasta, bread, and cereals. She cut out butter, margarine, mayonnaise, sauces, gravies, etc., altogether. She did not *ever* starve herself but would skip supper occasionally when she was too tired to eat.

This very high-quality real food regimen got her weight loss system going, and her body let go of forty pounds in the next six months! Karen's painstaking efforts to get and stay off the Feast-or-Famine Cycle for two years prior to this low-fat eating effort made it possible for her body to respond quickly to this important change in her diet.

Her body trusted her. She had been listening to its signals and feeding it well for two years, and her physiological need to keep fat was gone—naturally! The fat content in her diet was the key to the natural weight loss that followed. It's probably the key for many people.

Karen was happy with the loss that left her at 155 pounds and decided to add some fats and more red meats. She continued to eat when she felt really hungry but felt unconcerned and content when she experienced a little hunger. She let it go. In fact, she recalls that she was decidedly uninterested in eating at this point. Just like naturally thin people, Karen's life did not revolve around her diet anymore. She listed her favorite foods as raw fruits and vegetables, complex carbohydrates (cereal, pasta, breads), chicken, fish, and an occasional steak.

At this point Karen also ate hot dogs, hamburgers, and pizza when she was too tired or lazy to prepare higher-quality foods. She began to indulge in occasional chocolates, too, but without the cravings of her dieting days. Karen continued to lose weight on this more relaxed quality Anti-Diet and plateaued at 143, appearing thinner and better proportioned than when she began three years before.

Karen has been naturally thin at her ideal weight for over two years. Her weight fluctuates about four pounds with her menstrual cycle. She never diets. She eats freely whatever she wants whenever she wants to and has no fear of ever gaining weight again. She is content with her appetite and weight and feels pleased with her body. She is totally unafraid of eating, confident that her body can easily maintain a lean, naturally thin weight without her interference. Karen doesn't worry about not eating either, now that she and her body have learned to trust and take good care of each other.

Post recovery statistics: Karen, age 36

weight: 143-147 stable

recovery history: four years off Feast-or-Famine Cycle, two years at ideal weight

occupation: music teacher, domestic engineer

diet: quality real food eaten freely when hungry, no regular formal exercise, no binging, no overeating, no cravings for pleasure foods

cycle symptoms: none

recovery status: cured

effect of high predisposition to obesity: nearly three years to complete process of recovery to ideal weight, significant weight gain getting off Feast-or-Famine Cycle (complicated by pregnancy), required very strict high-quality (low-fat) Anti-Diet

eating program to stimulate initial weight loss
following year-long plateau

CASE #5 RAYA

Prerecovery statistics: Raya, age 8, female
weight: "chubby"
diet history: about one year
occupation: child, student
diet: trying to eat less, eating by external cues
   (watching and comparing others' eating to self),
   sneaking food and secret eating, parents' attempt
   to restrict diet
cycle symptoms: afraid and guilty about eating, preoccupied with food and eating, chronic undersatisfied hunger, anxious about food, feels out of
   control, poor body image (feels fat), weight gain
motive for recovery: pain of feeling fat and out of
   control, gradual increase in body fat causing worry
   and preoccupation with diet, wants to be "normal"
predisposition to obesity: mild (mild obesity in
   parent, none in siblings)

Raya's story is disturbing but not unusual. Exactly how
she first got on the Feast-or-Famine Cycle remains a
mystery. Maybe it was a normal chubby phase she went
through that caused her to begin to worry about eating.
Maybe it was our diet-crazed culture and skinny-body
insanity. Whatever led to her giving up ownership of her
diet, Raya was headed for a life-long struggle with
obesity at age 8.

One thing is certain: Raya's doctor contributed to the
problem. During a routine physical exam, Raya's doctor
told her to "cut down," referring of course to her eating.
That's all, just cut down. This is abusive and confusing to

an eight-year-old child. (It's confusing to me!) What does it mean? The doctor warned her that if she didn't cut down, she'd get fatter and fatter! I suppose this threat was meant to motivate Raya.

Had this particular doctor taken the time to find out about Raya's eating and worries about her weight, she would have discovered some disturbing facts. Raya was motivated to fix her weight problem. She was thinking about it all the time. And she was making many valiant efforts to control her eating, fighting her little body's instincts all the way. This doctor didn't need to threaten Raya with serious obesity. She needed to find the cause of Raya's cubbiness.

Unfortunately, medical doctors do not know much about obesity, and they are notoriously ill-equipped to help their patients with it. They still think obesity is caused by eating too much, period. They don't understand the Feast-or-Famine Cycle. And they would never tell an obese patient to stop dieting and eat more!

Luckily, Raya's story has a happy ending. Her mother shared her concern with me and took the Anti-Diet book home. She gave her daughter some basic sections to read and Raya asked her to copy the real-food lists. Raya grasped the Anti-Diet instantly. What a relief! She lost her fear of eating when she learned that *it* wasn't the problem. She stopped watching others eat and started tuning into her own hunger signals.

She got herself some real food to eat whenever she felt hungry and stopped eating when she felt full. Her parents stopped making suggestions or comments and let her have total ownership of her diet.

Emotionally, Raya was set free! She never thinks about food anymore, except when she gets hungry. And when she's really hungry and eats a lot, she doesn't feel guilty. She packs plenty of real food in her lunch box but often can't eat it all. She eats chips and sweets only occasionally, but doesn't worry about eating them, either.

Raya's body hasn't lost pounds and pounds, but she has had an enormous load of fear lifted. She has been relieved of the terrible fear of becoming fatter and fatter, unable to control or solve the problem. Raya understands what causes obesity, and she can be confident that she will never have to cope with it again. In a real sense, Raya has been restored to her childhood and the freedom children should all enjoy.

Post recovery statistics: Raya, age 9

weight: "firm"

recovery history: 18 months off Cycle, over one year at ideal weight

occupation: child, student

diet: eats real food on demand (by hunger), regular meals plus real food several times between, no parental involvement

cycle symptoms: none

recovery status: cured

effect of mild predisposition to obesity: fast adjustment getting off Feast-or-Famine Cycle, reached adaptive weight quickly

CASE #6 SNOWFLAKE

Prerecovery statistics: Snowflake the cat, age 7 months, female

weight: lean ideal (5.8 lbs.)

diet history: none until surgical interruption of food intake

occupation: pet

diet: high-quality cat food on demand (always available) until surgery

cycle symptoms: food withheld 12 hours before

surgery, unable to eat day of surgery (medically imposed famine), resumed feeding day after surgery and continued demand feeding which increased to overeating and weight gain for about two weeks, obviously overweight

motive for recovery: fat cats are not optimally healthy cats

predisposition to obesity: all domesticated animals are at risk for obesity

I like the way my vet determines the appropriateness of an animal's weight. He looks at the animal and feels its belly. You can see maladaptive fat, generally. He doesn't consult weight tables, partly because each animal is unique. Generalizations don't apply. This is true of people, too.

Snowflake was not on the Cycle for any period of time because she'd been on a demand feeding schedule since birth. Fortunately, it is recommended that kittens be fed on demand until about three months. Unfortunately, after that their food is restricted to some degree. Well, not my kitten. Naturally, we just kept feeding her high-quality cat food whenever she wanted it. We usually left enough food in her dish to ensure that she wouldn't get stranded hungry while we were out of the house.

Snowflake was at her ideal weight at seven months when we had her spayed. She looked lean and healthy and was active and energetic. I had heard the theory that spaying causes weight gain in female house pets, dooming them to life-long obesity. I was curious to see the effect that this surgery would have on Snowflake.

Her weight, recorded above, was taken before surgery. When we brought her home from the hospital, she appeared very thin and acted drowsy and weak. This is normal because of the anesthesia, interruption of food and fluids, and trauma of surgery.

We kept her food and water dishes full, and she regained her normal weight and appearance within a week or so. She was getting stronger and sleeping less. Gradually, I noticed that she was eating a lot and often, and she was getting fat! She had never been overweight before, but now her belly was becoming as round as a drum. She even waddled a bit!

Aha! Here it was—post-spay obesity! Right? Wrong! I never believed it either. Little Snowflake was just compensating for her week of "dieting", and I was confident that, with time and plenty of real food available, she would gradually get back to her slim self. And she did! We simply allowed her to eat as much real food (quality cat food) as she wanted whenever she got the urge. And in about three weeks she was looking sleek and slim again.

Snowflake is almost three years old now, and I've noticed that she tends to carry a little more weight during our cold Minnesota winters. She never looks fat, though, and the vet considers her adult weight perfect for her frame.

Post recovery statistics: Snowflake, age 3

weight: lean (9.6 pounds mature adult weight)

recovery history: two years off Cycle at ideal weight

occupation: pet

diet: eating pattern is erratic, always "asks" for food first thing in the morning, demand feeding high-quality cat food

cycle symptoms: none

recovery status: cured

effect of predisposition to obesity: three weeks to recover from just one five-day interruption in food availability, (overeating and fat storage in domestic animals who are food restricted is very efficient)

Point to ponder: What if I had decided to "help"

Snowflake lose her extra weight by putting her on a
little cat diet? Do you see how cats get fat from
spaying?

✣

GLOSSARY OF TERMS

adaptation—positive adjustment to environmental
influences

adaptive—promoting survival; supporting the life
and/or health of the organism and species

Anti-Diet—eating program which promotes body
regulation of food intake; permanent solution to
obesity that leads to gradual conversion of adaptive
obesity to adaptive (natural) lean by adjusting the
food availability of the environment

binge—eating unusually large amounts of food at one
time; overeating; eating without perception of
hunger; feast

borderline food—food containing significant nutrients but also having disproportionate amounts of
fats and/or sugars

diet—
  1) food ingested by an organism; what you eat
     (colloq.)
  2) attempt to lose weight by self-imposed food re-
     striction; basic cause of modern obesity

eating late—ingesting food more than fifteen minutes after hunger signals are first perceived

eating on time—ingesting food very soon after hunger signals are perceived

environment—surroundings of an organism

excessive hunger—physical perception of danger-
ously low body fuel accompanied by symptoms

which act as warning signals (i.e. headache, nausea, weakness, dizziness, irritability); stimulus for over-eating and high interest in fat-producing foods

famine—period of time when food is unavailable or available in insufficient quantities; eating amounts of food which do not satisfy hunger; undereating; eating avoidance; traditional low-calorie diet

feast—eating unusually large amounts of food at one time; overeating; binging; eating without perception of hunger

Feast-or-Famine Cycle—cyclic periods of undereating or semi-starvation followed by periods of overeating or binging; off and on dieting

food availability—level of quality ingestible nutrients available to be eaten without internal or external restriction

hunger—discomfort or drive associated with the physical need for food fuel

hunger signal—specific physical/mental communication of a food-fuel need

maladaptive—endangering survival; interfering with the life and/or health of the organism and species

naturally thin—maintaining a lean, adaptive body weight without significant conscious effort to regulate diet or eating behavior

obesity—maintenance of maladaptive amounts of fat in an environment of optimal food availability

pleasure food—food containing large amounts of fats and/or sugars; food typically low in nutrients; food designed mainly for taste satisfaction

quality food—food high in nutrient content and low in fats and sugars; real food

real food—food that meets body-fuel needs well; quality food

survival instinct—basic physiological drive to preserve your own life and the lives of offspring, powerful enough to override maladaptive choices in human beings

Theory of Adaptation—scientific concept describing how different species adjust to environmental influences in order to ensure the survival of the individual organism and species; basis for Anti-Diet concepts

variety food—foods representing all four traditional food groups

THE COMPLETE GUIDE TO A LIFETIME OF WELL-BEING BY AMERICA'S MOST TRUSTED HEALTH WRITER

JANE BRODY'S
The New York Times
— GUIDE TO —
PERSONAL HEALTH

Illustrated with graphs and charts, fully indexed and conveniently arranged under fifteen sections:

NUTRITION

EMOTIONAL HEALTH

ABUSED SUBSTANCES

EYES, EARS, NOSE AND THROAT

SAFETY

PESKY HEALTH PROBLEMS

COMMON KILLERS

EXERCISE

SEXUALITY AND REPRODUCTION

DENTAL HEALTH

ENVIRONMENTAL HEALTH EFFECTS

SYMPTOMS

COMMON SERIOUS ILLNESSES

MEDICAL CARE

COPING WITH HEALTH PROBLEMS

"Jane Brody's encyclopedia of wellness covers everything."
Washington Post

64121-6/$15.00 U.S./$18.00 Can.

Buy these books at your local bookstore or use this coupon for ordering:

Mail to: Avon Books, Dept BP, Box 767, Rte 2, Dresden, TN 38225   B
Please send me the book(s) I have checked above.
☐ My check or money order—no cash or CODs please—for $_____ is enclosed (please add $1.50 to cover postage and handling for each book ordered—Canadian residents add 7% GST).
☐ Charge my VISA/MC Acct#_____ Exp Date _____
Phone No _____ Minimum credit card order is $6.00 (please add postage and handling charge of $2.00 plus 50 cents per title after the first two books to a maximum of six dollars—Canadian residents add 7% GST). For faster service, call 1-800-762-0779. Residents of Tennessee, please call 1-800-633-1607. Prices and numbers are subject to change without notice. Please allow six to eight weeks for delivery.

Name _____

Address _____

City _____ State/Zip _____
                                                                JB 0892

Are you feeling OK about yourself?
Or still playing destructive games?
**THE 15-MILLION-COPY
NATIONAL BESTSELLER BY**
Thomas A. Harris, M.D.

I'M OK—
YOU'RE OK

00772-X/$4.95 US/$6.50 Can

**The Transactional Analysis Breakthrough that's
Changing the Consciousness and Behavior of People
Who Never Felt OK about Themselves.**

In *I'M OK—YOU'RE OK* find the freedom to change,
to liberate your adult effectiveness and to achieve a
joyful intimacy with the people in your life!

*And continue with a practical program for lifelong
well-being with*

STAYING OK
70130-8/$4.95 US/$5.95 Can

by Amy Bjork Harris
and Thomas A. Harris, M.D.

**on how to maximize good feelings, minimize bad ones,
and live life to the fullest!**

Buy these books at your local bookstore or use this coupon for ordering:

Mail to: Avon Books, Dept BP, Box 767, Rte 2, Dresden, TN 38225
Please send me the book(s) I have checked above.
☐ My check or money order—no cash or CODs please—for $_____ is enclosed
(please add $1.50 to cover postage and handling for each book ordered—Canadian
residents add 7% GST).
☐ Charge my VISA/MC Acct# _____ Exp Date _____
Phone No _____ Minimum credit card order is $6.00 (please add postage
and handling charge of $2.00 plus 50 cents per title after the first two books to a maximum
of six dollars—Canadian residents add 7% GST). For faster service, call 1-800-762-0779.
Residents of Tennessee, please call 1-800-633-1607. Prices and numbers are subject to
change without notice. Please allow six to eight weeks for delivery.

Name _____
Address _____
City _____ State/Zip _____

OK 0892